AIDS AND THE
NEW ORPHANS

AIDS AND THE NEW ORPHANS

COPING WITH DEATH

Edited by Barbara O. Dane and Carol Levine

Foreword by Barbara Blum

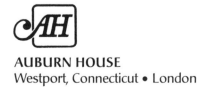

AUBURN HOUSE
Westport, Connecticut • London

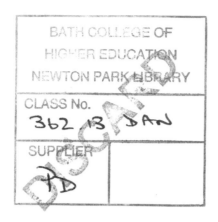
Library of Congress Cataloging-in-Publication Data

AIDS and the new orphans : coping with death / edited by Barbara O.
   Dane and Carol Levine ; foreword by Barbara Blum.
      p. cm.
   Includes bibliographical references and index.
   ISBN 0–86569–220–3.—ISBN 0–86569–249–1 (pbk.)
    1. Children of AIDS patients. 2. Bereavement.   I. Dane, Barbara
O. II. Levine, Carol.
   RA644.A25A3537   1994
   362.1'969792—dc20   94–4755

British Library Cataloguing in Publication Data is available.

Library of Congress Catalog Card Number: 94–4755
ISBN: 0–86569–220–3
    0–86569–249–1 (pbk.)

First published in 1994

Auburn House, 88 Post Road West, Westport, CT 06881
An imprint of Greenwood Publishing Group, Inc.

Printed in the United States of America

The paper used in this book complies with the
Permanent Paper Standard issued by the National
Information Standards Organization (Z39.48–1984).

10 9 8 7 6 5 4 3 2 1

Contents

Foreword

The cataclysmic but still largely hidden impacts of AIDS on America's children is examined carefully and constructively in the chapters of this book. The authors of *AIDS and the New Orphans: Coping with Death* have collaborated skillfully to create a knowledge base drawn from what we know about the development of children, about bereavement, and about HIV/AIDS. The integration of this knowledge allows the reader to develop a fresh, albeit sobering, perspective on the scale and nature of problems faced by orphaned children.

The Centers for Disease Control and Prevention is quoted in the first chapter as stating that "the recognition of a disease and its emergence as a leading cause of death within the same decade is without precedent." The slowness of our response to the effects of this disease has contributed to its impact on children, 80 percent of them from minority families. While coping with parental loss has always strained the capacity of family members and community institutions, children orphaned by AIDS present new and greater challenges. The stigma attached to AIDS and the developmental and cultural variations in responding to death are clearly delineated and provide us with an informed understanding about ways to meet those challenges.

What comes clear throughout this volume is the central role that family relationships play in dealing with the tragedy of death from AIDS. The orphan, whether HIV-infected or uninfected, is best supported when there are family members willing and able to provide a stable home. As in so many circumstances affecting children, the need for continuity must be recognized and valued, whatever the developmental stage of the child.

One must ask, then, how family members can be supported so that the children of parents with AIDS can benefit from familial care. To answer that question, support systems need to be designed using the cultural underpinnings of the families themselves. That means that there cannot be a single "program" intervention, a panacea that is so frequently sought by policymakers. Rather, as the authors adroitly point out, the strengths that exist within the family's community, through religion, and from intrafamily dynamics need, in each case, to be marshaled to respond to each individual situation.

The authors have developed the case for major and dramatic changes in public policy and in human service practice to ameliorate the tragedies faced by tens of thousands of America's children. Policymakers and practitioners should take heed.

Barbara Blum
President
Foundation for Child Development

1

The New Orphans and Grieving in the Time of AIDS

Carol Levine

Some human catastrophes announce themselves with unmistakable fury: natural disasters like earthquakes, volcano eruptions, and floods; techno-logical disasters like the chemical explosions in Bhopal, India, or the nuclear meltdown at Chernobyl in the Ukraine; and medical disasters like a cholera epidemic.

But human disasters also arrive not with a bang but a whimper, to paraphrase T. S. Eliot. The epidemic of the acquired immunodeficiency syndrome (AIDS) officially began slowly, almost imperceptibly. In the United States the signal event was the report of the Centers for Disease Control and Prevention (CDC) in June 1981 that in Los Angleles, extremely rare cases of *Pneumocystis carinii* pneumonia (PCP) had been diagnosed in five previously healthy homosexual men, two of whom had died (CDC 1981a). This was not, of course, the actual beginning. One month later the CDC reported that since January 1979, 26 homosexual men in New York City and California had been diagnosed with Kaposi's sarcoma. Many had also been diagnosed with PCP and other viral diseases; eight had died (CDC 1981b). In August 1981 the CDC reported that five heterosexuals, including one woman, had been diagnosed with similar conditions related to the severe immune deficiency now called AIDS or, in Spanish, SIDA (CDC 1986, 2–4).

In the second decade of the epidemic, in an odd congruence of meanings, the statistics (the "numbers") of people dead and dying from this disease are in truth numbing. In the United States alone, as of the end of July 1993, the CDC reported that 315,390 men, women, and children had been diag-nosed with AIDS (the end stage of HIV, or human immunodeficiency virus, disease). Of this total, 310,680 were adults or adolescents over the age of 13, and 4,710 were children under the age of 13. Death has taken a heavy toll: 61.7 percent (191,824) of the adults had died, as had 53.3 percent (2,510) of the children (CDC 1993a).

In reviewing the fifteen leading causes of death in the United States for 1989, the CDC noted the sharp increase—33 percent from the previous year—in deaths related to HIV infection. "The recognition of a disease and its emergence as a leading cause of death within the same decade is without precedent," the normally laconic CDC commented (CDC 1992a). Nearly three quarters of these deaths occurred among men and women aged 25 to 44. For this age group nationally HIV infection is the second leading cause of death for men and the sixth for women. In 1990 and 1991, this age group's death rates for most other leading causes of death declined or remained relatively stable, but the death rate for HIV infection steadily increased (CDC 1993c).

AIDS cases among women were reported almost from the beginning. But because of the overwhelming impact on gay men, especially white gay men, and the government's and the media's almost singleminded focus on this population in the early years, AIDS as a threat to women and children was underestimated. Yet AIDS is already the leading cause of death among African-American women aged 15 to 44 in New York City (New York City Department of Health 1989). While 9 percent of the first 100,000 persons with AIDS were women, women constituted 12 percent of the second 100,000, and the proportion of women among all persons with AIDS will continue to rise (CDC 1992b). Almost half of the women with AIDS nationally have been injecting drug users, and an additional fifth were infected through heterosexual contact with infected drug users (CDC 1993a). The proportion infected heterosexually continues to rise; in 1992, for the first time, the number of AIDS cases among women infected through heterosexual contact exceeded the number of those infected through injection drug use (CDC 1993b). The increase in cases among women should come as no surprise, for in many other nations where AIDS has gained momentum, the numbers of infected men and women have been nearly equal.

Because AIDS among women has been strongly associated with injecting drug use, endemic in poor communities of color, the majority of infected women have come from these already devastated urban centers. In their families, women are the primary caregivers. When they die, they leave children of all ages, some of whom need shelter, food, and medical care, and all of whom need emotional support and guidance.

ESTIMATES OF NUMBERS OF ORPHANED YOUTH

Just as AIDS took the nation (and the world) by surprise, AIDS among women took far too long to be recognized as a serious problem in the United States. From the first five cases reported to the CDC in 1981 to the millions of cases of HIV infection estimated by the World Health Organization (WHO) today, epidemiologists have tried to quantify almost all aspects of the rising tide of the AIDS epidemic. Even though the epidemic has hit hard at women and men in their prime reproductive years, only in the past few years has a basic question been raised: How many children and adolescents will survive the death of a parent of an HIV-related cause?

People living and working in the hardest hit communities have known many families with surviving children, but there was no epidemiologic model to estimate their actual number. The Orphan Project, as one of its first tasks, developed such a model for New York City and the United States (Michaels and Levine 1992). It then applied this model to five other cities: Newark, Miami, San Juan, Los Angeles, and Washington, DC.[1]

The various categories of children and adolescents who are infected with or affected by HIV can be represented schematically in the form of an iceberg. The tip of the iceberg represents the nearly 5,000 pediatric AIDS cases in the United States reported to the CDC (including the small but growing number of reported adolescent cases). Understandably, pediatric AIDS has received the most public and professional attention, since these fragile children and their families have urgent medical and social service needs. Just below the tip of the iceberg, and only partially visible above the water line, are known cases of HIV-infected children and adolescents. That there are many more HIV-infected newborns than known pediatric AIDS cases—more than three times as many in 1989, for example (Oxtoby 1991)—means that a large portion of this section of the iceberg is still hidden.

The next largest portion of the iceberg represents the uninfected siblings of the group with AIDS or HIV infection. These may be older brothers and sisters, born before their mother contracted HIV, or younger children who escaped maternal-fetal transmission. Current rates of maternal-fetal transmission in the New York City area range from 20 to 30 percent—lower than those in Africa but considerably higher than those in Europe, for still unexplained reasons (Boylan and Stein 1991).

By far the largest and most hidden portion of the iceberg lies at its base. This portion includes uninfected children and adolescents for whom a parent or parents, another adult relative, or a person unrelated by birth or marriage who has by commitment and loyalty come to be considered family has either died of AIDS or is living with AIDS or serious HIV disease. To carry the image one step further, the iceberg itself is situated in a stormy sea of violence, homelessness, drug and alcohol use, poverty, discrimination, and community disintegration.

Although in recent years the term "orphan" has been used most commonly to describe a child who has lost both parents, throughout Western history it has been used to define a child who has lost one or both parents. A definition that focuses on motherless youth was chosen for this epidemiological model, partly because such a definition conforms to the realities of life as these families know it. For the vast majority of youth whose caregiving parent dies of HIV, that parent is the mother. There are, of course, families in which an HIV-infected father is the primary caregiver; however, these situations appear to be rare. There are also families in which the death of the father from AIDS, even when the mother is uninfected, is a traumatic event that results in breakup of the family. Although these scenarios are important in developing programs to meet the range of individual needs, as described in later chapters, they do not affect the broad epidemiological picture.

The definition also conforms to the realities of epidemiological analysis, because there are few data on the offspring of men dying of HIV disease. For these reasons, this definition is used by the CDC (Caldwell et al. 1992), WHO, and the United Nations Children's Emergency Fund (UNICEF 1991, 5–6). If data on fathers were available, it would be possible to estimate the number of children who will lose their fathers to the epidemic, which would dramatically increase the number of children reported here. However, there are no statistics available for men that are the equivalent of fertility rates among women. Because no one has calculated the general rate at which men father children, it is impossible to estimate how many children will be left fatherless because of HIV. Even so, a series of studies of selected populations of men (in drug treatment centers, for example) would provide data to illuminate this important question.

HIV has come to rival or surpass other important causes of death in taking the lives of mothers of young children nationally. Among women under the age of 50, cancer is the cause of death of mothers of approximately 4,200 children and 8,700 adolescents annually. Motor vehicle accidents are responsible for the deaths of mothers of an additional 3,200 children and 1,900 adolescents. By contrast, the numbers of children and adolescents annually left motherless by HIV are predicted to reach 3,900 and 3,400, respectively, by 1994.

Figure 1 shows three estimates of children and adolescents left mother-less by HIV, based on a range of values for the proportions of HIV-related deaths identified on death certificates, the pediatric AIDS and overall infant mortality rates, the number of projected AIDS deaths among women in the future, and other parameters used in the model. Unless the course of the epidemic changes dramatically, by the year 2000, the overall number of motherless children and adolescents in the United States will exceed 80,000, with a range of 72,000 to 125,000. More than 40,000 of these will be children under 12 years old, and more than 30,000 will be adolescents between the ages of 13 and 17. In 1991, more than 80 percent of all youth whose mothers died of HIV/AIDS–related complications were offspring of African-American or Hispanic children (Michaels and Levine 1992).

Using a different model, the CDC arrived at a similar estimate, predicting that between 93,000 and 112,000 children will be born to mothers who die

Figure 1
Motherless Children & Adolescents Orphaned by HIV/AIDS, U.S.
Cumulative, 1981–2000

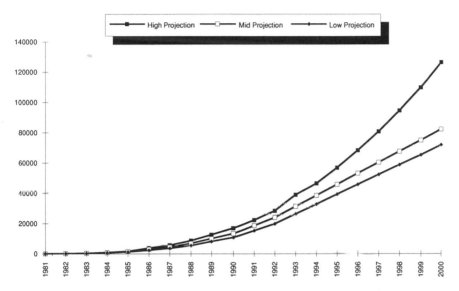

Source: From Chapter 1, by Carol Levine and Gary L. Stein, *Orphans of the HIV Epidemic: Unmet Needs in Six U.S. Cities* (New York: The Orphan Project, 1994).

of HIV between 1992 and the year 2000. Additionally, these women will give birth to between 32,000 and 38,000 children infected with HIV during the decade (Caldwell et al. 1992).

The existence of a large number of orphaned youngsters can no longer be ignored. Meeting their needs, and those of their families, will require the combined efforts of many people and agencies (Levine 1993). It is important, as a start, to look at the context in which these efforts toward assisting in bereavement will take place.

HOW COMMUNITIES REACT AND RESPOND TO DEATHS

"Communities" are not easily defined or categorized; they are made up of unique individuals with varying degrees of similarity. Yet certain generalizations can be made about their response to AIDS.

In gay communities, the AIDS epidemic followed a short but intense period of sexual freedom and expression in the 1970s. For many gay men this was the first time in their lives that they felt whole as individuals, no longer forced to conceal their sexual orientation. The grief and dismay that followed death after death were linked not only to the staggering loss of friends and lovers but also to the loss of sexual freedom or at least sexual freedom without fear of death. A period of unparalleled joy and exuberance was followed by one of unrelenting pain and mourning.

Despite a general relaxation of moralistic attitudes about sexuality, including homosexuality, many gay men had not "come out" to their parents or other family members. They lived in at least two different worlds: a gay world where they associated primarily with gay men and lesbians, and the straight world of their birth. More than a few gay men were forced to tell their unknowing parents that they were both gay and dying. In some cases the two worlds mixed on special occasions, but rarely were they fully integrated. For gay men who also belonged to an ethnic or religious minority—Latino or African-American or Irish or Jewish—the straight world was itself split into the mainstream culture and the minority culture of their families and earliest friends.

The growth of a powerful sense of community and the beginnings of political organization in the halcyon days of the 1960s and 1970s made it possible for gay men to mobilize quickly to create gay-directed organizations, educational programs, and services for their sick comrades. These activities not only filled the void of nonexistent mainstream services, but they also provided a meaningful outlet to turn grief about one's losses and anxiety about one's own health into positive actions to help friends and community members. The Gay Men's Health Crisis in New York City, formed in 1981 by a few men who came together for self-education, is now the city's largest private social service agency, utilizing hundreds of volunteers (Ouellette Kobasa 1991). Organizations with political goals, for example, ACT UP, provided an activist alternative for volunteers.

Many gay men created and used distinctive rituals around death in positive and innovative ways. The most dramatic and powerful example is undoubtedly the Names Project, created by Cleve Jones of San Francisco. Inspired by the folk traditions of quilting and sewing bees, the Names Project's AIDS Memorial Quilt is made up of thousands of panels, each memorializing a man, woman, or child who has died of AIDS. These tangible and highly personal tributes—some humorous, some elegant, some simple—stand as eloquent witness to the lives lost in the epidemic. Other common rituals include the release of balloons after a memorial service to symbolize the soul's liberation from the body's pain, funeral services and wakes carefully planned by the dying patient, the lighting of candles in marches or silent memorials. While religion has played a part, even a major part, in some funerals, often the service or memorial is devoid of traditional religious ceremonies.

The devastation of the epidemic in gay communities has been captured in literature, art, music, and drama. These expressive forms offer a catharsis for audiences in the original Greek sense in which theater was a purging of emotions. There are many examples: John Corigliano's *Symphony No. 1*, Paul Monette's novels, plays by Tony Kushner and Larry Kramer, dances by Bill T. Jones, photographs by Nicholas Nixon, paintings by Ross Bleckner, and literally dozens of other works. Although many of the works are somber, humor also plays a large role in catharsis, for example, in the play *Falsettoland* by William Finn. "Cancer has killed more people but has engendered virtually no art," wrote critic Michael Kimmelman in 1989. "One must struggle to think of an art form that has not been affected by AIDS" (Kimmelman 1989).

While the cumulative impact of multiple losses in the gay community has been enormous, the community's response has helped alleviate the pain. One study of over 200 gay men in New York City found an unexpectedly small number of depressive disorders and depressive symptoms. While acknowledging these results as preliminary, the authors suggest that "the gay community has developed effective coping mechanisms to assist members in dealing with multiple losses" (Neugebauer et al. 1992).

The response to AIDS deaths in African-American and Latino communities, where the majority of surviving children live, has differed in ways that significantly affect expressions of grief. Repeating the caveat that "communities" are made up of many individuals with varying beliefs and characteristics, some generalizations can be offered.

The advent of AIDS coincided with a period in which communities of color were struggling with the results of a century of neglect, discrimination, and poverty. Unlike the mainstream gay community, which was embarking on community building, African-American and Latino communities were witnessing disintegration. AIDS, and its link to drug use as well as homosexuality, was seen not as *the* major disaster threatening community existence (as it was among gay populations) but as just one more misery to add to a long list of unaddressed problems. A longstanding distrust of government, and especially of public health agencies, has led to support for theories that AIDS was a man-made disease created to destroy communities of color. Official explanations of the cause of disease and programs to combat it are often seen as part of a conspiracy of genocide (Thomas and Quinn 1991).

With very few exceptions in the early years, community leaders did not mobilize around AIDS and give the epidemic the benefit of their prestige and support. As a result, the mainstream stigma of AIDS was not counterbalanced by community attitudes but in fact was reinforced by them. This situation has begun to change in the past several years, as more African-American and Latino leaders and organizations have addressed their communities' needs for education and services. For example, in 1993 the National Baptist Convention, USA, announced at its convention that 750 churches have been enlisted to serve on black leadership coalitions on AIDS in 17 cities (Polner 1993).

Unlike gay communities in which early death had been a rarity before AIDS, dying young was commonplace in communities of color. Young adults died frequently of drug use, violence, or inadequate medical care. AIDS added another potential cause of death, but it did not require a quantum leap to comprehend the possibility that young people might die.

Communities of color already had traditions and rituals around death. They did not need to create a new and distinctive way of expressing grief as did gay communities. But funerals and wakes that used these traditions often maintained the veil of secrecy that had surrounded the illness, thus compounding the stigma. A diagnosis that had to be hidden in life could not be acknowledged in death. In some instances, even the traditional rituals and practices had to be curtailed because of funeral directors' reluctance to handle the body, religious leaders' condemnation of the sexual or drug-using behaviors that preceded the death, or the family's wish to downplay the death.

Again with a few exceptions, the extraordinarily rich talent of African-American and Latino artists and writers has not found expression around AIDS. Other themes have predominated. Even where AIDS has been presented in artistic forms (notably drama), the purpose has been didactic, that is, to educate people about risk reduction or the benefits of early medical intervention. Some gay men of color have created artistic works, but these have emphasized their gay experience, rather than their cultural roots. The lack of a body of artistic work that acts as a catharsis for a community has reinforced stigma and secrecy.

Richard Goldstein, a writer and critic, comments:

The arts enabled gay men to bear witness to their situation, express feelings of grief that society often distorts, and create a model for communal solidarity, personal devotion, and sexual caution. . . . No comparable process of self-expression exists among the other groups hit hardest by AIDS—IV drug users, their children, and their mostly black or Hispanic partners—in part because there is no "community" perceived as such, to bind drug users together. In their isolation and secrecy, these people with AIDS are far less visible than the middle-class white homosexuals whose plight has been so amply documented. (Goldstein 1991, p. 19)

The cumulative effects of all these factors on surviving family members have been avoidance, shame, and guilt. These attitudes are communicated to children either explicitly or implicitly. As a result, opportunities to grieve in appropriate ways and to be supported in these expressions are few. Yet there is enormous potential to build on the existing cultural and religious heritage to create meaningful modes of expression that allow children to feel not only their loss but also the support of their own community and, ultimately, the support of the larger community as well.

This support and other similar efforts will come from those who are affected by AIDS and who look to the future and see a generation of children grieving for a generation of lost parents.

IN THESE PAGES

This book represents the individual and collective efforts of a group of professionals involved in the fields of bereavement, AIDS, or children. Recognizing that the literature on each of these issues is very rich, and that the literature on any two is extensive, but that the literature that addresses all three is very sparse, the editors asked a number of colleagues to address the complex interrelationships in these three subjects. Their efforts are represented in this book. Because there are very few specific research findings to draw upon, many of the chapters are based on casework experience and research from related fields. Much more research needs to be done to explore fully the themes of isolation, stigma, and "disenfranchised" grief (to use Kenneth Doka's telling phrase) that pervade these pages.

Barbara Dane sets the stage for the succeeding chapters by presenting an analysis of how Western culture approaches death, demonstrating that avoidance of discussion of AIDS deaths must be understood in the cultural context of denial of death in general.

For surviving children and their new guardians, death is not the end but the beginning. Kenneth Doka provides an expansive vision of spirituality and children, going beyond religious beliefs and institutional structures to reach the hearts and souls of children and their beliefs about death and dead parents. The next two chapters explore the issues of childhood bereavement related to AIDS from the perspective of age and developmental stage. Karolynn Siegel and Barbara Freund look at latency-age children, and Luis Zayas and Kathleen Romano describe adolescents.

These chapters are followed by two analyses of the role of culture and ethnicity in understanding AIDS-related bereavement. Esther Chachkes and Regina Jennings portray Latino cultural patterns that influence bereavement, and Lucretia Phillips and Penelope Johnson-Moore describe the black community's response. Gary Anderson analyzes the conflicts and problems that new guardians face as they attempt to build a new and secure relationship with grieving youngsters. Finally, Diane Grodney describes four projects that are reaching children and families and gives valuable recommendations to practitioners.

Practitioners and other professionals, like the families they serve, also grieve. Our losses, while not as deep as those felt by intimates, are nonetheless real and cumulative. We too need to acknowledge grief and permit healing. By acknowledging our own losses, we help children come to terms with theirs. By attending to children's grief, we assuage our own.

NOTE

1. The following section is based on the work of David Michaels, Ph.D., M.P.H., associate professor of epidemiology in the Department of Community Health and Social Medicine at the City University of New York Medical School/Sophie Davis School of Biomedical Education, New York City. The analysis appears in slightly different form in David Michaels and Carol Levine, "The Youngest Survivors: Estimates of the Number of Youth Orphaned by AIDS in New York City," in Carol Levine, ed., *A Death in the Family: Orphans of the HIV Epidemic* (New York: United Hospital Fund, 1993), pp. 3–12 and in Chapter 1, Carole Levine and Gary L. Stein, *Orphans of the HIV Epidemic: Unmet Needs in Six U.S. Cities* (New York: The Orphan Project, 1994).

REFERENCES

Boylan, Laura, and Zena A. Stein. 1991. "The Epidemiology of HIV Infection in Children and Their Mothers: Vertical Transmission." *Epidemiologic Reviews* 13:143–177.

Caldwell, M. Blake, P.L. Fleming, and Maragaret J. Oxtoby. 1992. "Estimated Number of AIDS Orphans in the United States." *Pediatrics* 90:482.

Centers for Disease Control. 1981a. "Pneumocystis Pneumonia—Los Angeles." *Morbidity and Mortality Weekly Report* 30:250–252.

———. 1981b. "Kaposi's Sarcoma and Pneumocystis Pneumonia among Homosexual Men—New York City and California." *Morbidity and Mortality Weekly Report* 30:305–307.

———. 1986. *Reports on AIDS Published in the Morbidity and Mortality Weekly Report, June 1981 through February 1986.* Springfield, VA: National Technical Information Service.

———. 1992a. "Mortality Patterns—United States, 1989." *Morbidity and Mortality Weekly Report* 41:121–125.

———. 1992b. "The Second 100,000 Cases of Acquired Immunodeficiency Syndrome." *Morbidity and Mortality Weekly Report* 41:28–29.

———. 1993a. *HIV/AIDS Surveillance Report* Second Quarter Edition 5(2):3, 12.

———. 1993b. "Update: Acquired Immunodeficiency Syndrome—United States, 1992." *Morbidity and Mortality Weekly Report* 42:551, 557.

———. 1993c. "Update: Mortality Attributable to HIV Infection/AIDS Among Persons Aged 25–44 Years—United States, 1990 and 1991." *Morbidity and Mortality Weekly Report* 42:481–486.

Eliot, T. S. 1930. "The Hollow Men." In *Selected Poems.* San Diego, CA: Harcourt Brace Jovanovich.

Goldstein, Richard. 1991. "The Implicated and the Immune: Responses to AIDS in the Arts and Popular Culture." In *A Disease of Society: Cultural & Institutional Responses to AIDS*, eds. Dorothy Nelkin, David P. Willis, and Scott V. Parris, 17–42. New York: Cambridge University Press.

Kimmelman, Michael. 1989. "Bitter Harvest: AIDS and the Arts." *The New York Times* (19 March) Section 2, p. 1.

Levine, Carol, ed. 1993. *A Death in the Family: Orphans of the HIV Epidemic*. New York: United Hospital Fund.

Levine, Carol, and Gary L. Stein. 1994. *Orphans of the HIV Epidemic: Unmet Needs in Six U.S. Cities*. New York: The Orphan Project.

Michaels, David, and Carol Levine. 1992. "Estimates of the Number of Motherless Youth Orphaned by AIDS in the United States." *Journal of the American Medical Association* 268:3456–3461.

Neugebauer, Richard, Judith Rabkin, Janet B.W. Williams, Robert H. Remien, Raymond Goetz, and Jack M. Gorman. 1992. "Bereavement Reactions Among Homosexual Men Experiencing Multiple Losses in the AIDS Epidemic." *American Journal of Psychiatry* 149:1374–1379.

New York City Department of Health. 1989. *Summary of Vital Statistics, 1989*.

Ouellette Kobasa, Suzanne C. 1991. "AIDS Volunteering: Links to the Past and Future Prospects." In *A Disease of Society: Cultural & Institutional Responses to AIDS*, eds. Dorothy C. Nelkin, David P. Willis, and Scott V. Paris, 172–188. New York: Cambridge University Press.

Oxtoby, Margaret J. 1991. "Perinatally Acquired HIV Infection." In *Pediatric AIDS*, eds. P. A. Pizzo and Catherine M. Wilfert, 9–10. Baltimore, MD: Williams & Wilkins.

Polner, Rob. 1993. "Baptists Plan Tactics in War Against AIDS." *New York Newsday* (6 September).

Thomas, Stephen B., and Sandra Crouse Quinn. 1991. "The Tuskegee Syphilis Study, 1932 to 1972: Implications for HIV Education and AIDS Risk Education Programs in the Black Community." *American Journal of Public Health* 81:1498–1505.

United Nations Children's Fund. 1991. *Report on a Meeting About AIDS and Orphans in Africa, Florence 14/15 June 1991*. New York: United Nations Children's Fund.

2

Death and Bereavement

Barbara O. Dane

Bereavement clearly ranks high among stressful life events (Sanders 1980; Holmes and Rahe 1967). The loss of a cherished and significant relationship can have both overt and inner psychological effects. As with other human behavior, reaction to loss can be expressed in many ways. To introduce more specific chapters on the grief children and adolescents experience as they cope with a parent's death from AIDS, this chapter will discuss general responses to death and bereavement. Six salient features of an AIDS death that can influence grieving will be presented to help mental health clinicians improve the effectiveness of their interventions. They are (1) overall cultural responses to death and the mourning process; (2) socially unspeakable death, which tends to carry stigma, fear of contagion, discrimination, and secrecy; (3) relationship to the deceased; (4) the child's and adolescent's understanding of death; (5) survivor guilt; and (6) social supports.

OVERVIEW OF CULTURAL ATTITUDES TOWARD DEATH AND GRIEF

In order to appreciate a person's attitude toward death, a wide range of variables should be considered: that person's social, cultural, religious, philosophical, and ethnic background. Different cultures view death and dying and the practices or rituals associated with them from multiple perspectives based on education, socioeconomic status, and religious beliefs. Each society's response to death is influenced by its teleological view of life. There seem to be two general cultural patterns of response to death: death-accepting and death-denying.

Greek folk tradition, for example, accepts the finality of death. Acceptance is expressed in laments (Dracopoulou and Doxiadis 1988):

When should I expect you? Until when should I wait for you? Until the sea runs dry and becomes a garden, until the crow turns white and becomes a dove. Expect me then. Wait for me until then. (Petropoulos 1959, p. 223)

Five years after death, the bones of the deceased are exhumed by relatives and friends, washed in wine, and put in the village ossuary. This ritual symbolizes the realization that the deceased will never return (Danforth 1982, 15–23; 48–69).

American Indian ritual provides another example of a death-accepting culture. In her poignant short story, "The Man to Send Rain Clouds," the Laguna Pueblo writer Leslie Silko (1974) describes the events at the end of the old man Teofilo's life. When his children find him dead at a sheep camp, they paint his face and tie a small feather in his hair. There is a smile on his son's face as he strews corn meal and pollen in the wind and bids his father to send rain clouds. This aspect of the funeral rite of passage reveals the Pueblo people's belief in the interdependence of the living and the dead. If one lives a proper life into old age, one will become a cloud or kachina spirit in death. For many cultures in North America, the journey along life's road does not end in death but continues beyond this world.

In comparison with many cultures, Western cultures restrict the expression of grief. The United States has epitomized a death-denying culture. Death, perhaps humanity's greatest mystery, has become increasingly distant from everyday life. Although we recognize the universality of death—even our personal destiny to die simply because we were born—death is kept at a distance, remote, and impersonal. Thinking or talking about death is regarded as morbid. Health and youth are idealized; illness and old age are devalued. Most deaths take place out of view in nursing homes and hospitals. This denial of death makes it more frightening and difficult to face. Nevertheless, because of the expected and predictable nature of death among the elderly, Western culture has been structured to prepare for the event, and certain coping mechanisms are available to survivors after such deaths.

As Freud and others (Lifton 1979; Segal 1988; Meissner 1988) have suggested, denial is a universal adaptation to the threat of personal death, that is, annihilation. World War I disillusioned Freud. He was horrified by the eradication of the rules of civilized moral and social conduct and the brutality with which men could inflict death and suffering upon other human beings (Freud 1968). His answer was psychological denial of personal death:

Our own death is indeed unimaginable, . . . at bottom no one believes in his own death, or to put the same thing in another way, in the unconscious every one of us is convinced of his own immortality. (Freud, as quoted in Rickman 1968, p. 15).

Ernest Becker (1973) agreed. He wrote, "This narcissim is what keeps men marching into point-blank fire in wars: at heart one doesn't feel he will die, he only feels sorry for the man next to him" (p. 2). Lifton (1979) observes:

And our resistance to that knowledge, our denial of death, is indeed formidable. . . . But the denial can never be total; we are never fully ignorant of the fact that we die. Rather we go about life with a kind of "middle knowledge" of death, a partial awareness of it side by side with expressions and actions that belie that awareness. (p. 17)

Although death is generally viewed as uncontrollable and undesirable, Marshall (1980) suggests that some people find it preferable to mental deterioration; feelings of uselessness, pain and suffering; and being a burden. It is not unusual for people to say that they would not want to live with the degree of impairment of the dying person with AIDS or other diseases.

The denial and externalization of death, which have been so characteristic of twentieth-century Western society, have eroded somewhat in the past few decades through the popularization of the "Death and Dying" educational movement. Adolescents and children are learning once again that death is a part of what it means to be human, and that it is inhumane for people to die all alone, attached to tubes and life-sustaining machines, without being given a chance to make their peace and say their good-byes.

THE MOURNING PROCESS

The literature on the nature of grief and bereavement has been growing ever since the publication of Lindemann's (1944) classic article, "Symptomatology and Management of Acute Grief." Most of the literature has focused on grief reactions of a parent, spouse, or child. For example, Glick et al. (1974), Bowling and Cartwright (1982), and Parkes and Weiss (1983) have provided comprehensive studies of grief reactions. Palombo (1981), in discussing the loss of a love object through death, describes the process as characterized by initial shock, disbelief (especially if the death is unexpected), and denial. Volkan (1972) provides a detailed description of atypical manifestations of grief.

Kubler-Ross (1969) stressed the importance of treating death as a natural part of life. With each loss we search to replace, restore, and readapt to the changes brought on by the break in our attachment to the object or person.

We grieve for our losses, whether loss of home, social networks, routines, surroundings, possessions, or the ultimate loss of a parent through death.

Hoagland (1984) points out that one of the most important discoveries about bereavement is that the symptoms tend to follow a predictable course over time. One must go through grief work, grieving for one's losses (or sometimes multiple losses as in AIDS deaths) in order to heal the wounds. When the wound is healed, there will be a scar, but it will be a healed psychological wound.

Bowlby and Parkes (1979) describe four phases of the mourning process: (1) shock and numbness, (2) yearning and searching, (3) disorientation and disorganization, and (4) resolution and reorganization. All four dimensions are usually present when the mourner learns of the death. There are highs and lows in the process and no neat dividing lines between the characteristics. As the mourner begins to resolve conflicts of the loss, feelings of shock and numbness pass; there is less searching and yearning. Disorientation and disorganization appear less frequently, and the mourner reorganizes to learn how to relate to the world without the deceased. It is the resolution of the conflicts brought on by the death, not the passage of time, by which the mourner achieves resolution of the process. Time alone does not heal. For those who avoid grief work, time does nothing but pass, leaving grievers to deal with unresolved, delayed grief reactions, which may become exaggerated and complicated. Grief work may dominate the life of the mourner since it takes time to resolve the many changes in one's life brought about by the death of a loved one.

Contemporary models of grief are largely based on the attachment model. The concept of attachment (Bowlby 1980) refers to the tendency of individuals to make lasting bonds of affection with others and accounts for the emotional responses that result when these bonds are disrupted, threatened with separation, or permanently lost.

SOCIALLY UNACCEPTABLE DEATH

Until recently, little research (Dane and Miller 1992; Doka 1987; Geis et al. 1986; Peppers and Knapp 1980) has been directed to grief reactions in socially unrecognized or stigmatized grief. Although each surviving orphan had a unique relationship with the deceased parent, he or she will experience the death and grief differently. Stigmatized grievers keep their grief, guilt, shame, and anger locked inside. In the case of an AIDS death, survivors are doubly disenfranchised. There are no models or culturally prescribed roles for AIDS mourners in our society, making it even more difficult for children and adolescents to grieve successfully.

Bereavement reactions of children and adolescents are very strongly influenced by the dynamics of social attitudes prior to parental death and the dynamics of the grieving process itself. To understand better how children and adolescents react to parental death, it is esssential to examine the struggle of living with the fear, anger, and rejection that persons with AIDS and their survivors experience. The physical and psychological systems of the person may be overwhelmed by the demands placed on them. This often leads to physical distress and feelings of helplessness and depression.

Death from AIDS, like death from suicide, profoundly alters survivors' social relationships as a consequence of real or imagined stigma. A stigma is a mark of shame or discredit. Stigmatization is a belief in and internalization of negative attitudes, resulting in a redefinition of the self as worthy of hatred and rejection. This redefinition occurs not only for the reference group but for the self as well. The focus of social psychological research on stigma is not on the mark itself, however, so much as on the social relationships in which a particular mark is defined as shameful or discrediting (Goffman 1963).

Survivors responding to Rudestam's (1977) survey on suicide indicated that they felt unprepared and described the event as being "like a devastating emotional blow" (p. 222). Like those who survive a loved one's death from suicide, secondary AIDS survivors experience trauma, shame, guilt, insecurity, and disorientation. There is also a tendency for survivors to deny, avoid, retreat, isolate, and wish to escape. They experience intensely negative reactions that shape their behavior and limit their effectiveness in achieving a healthy outcome to their grieving.

Parents with AIDS, like other people with AIDS, and their children experience and witness diverse psychosocial stressors including social ostracism, rejection, and isolation; radically altered roles; loss of control over and destruction of expectations for the future; and fear of physical and mental disability (Dane 1990; Forstein 1984; Morin et al. 1984). Survivors must bear the burden of societal hostility at a time when they are most in need of social support. Fears of shame and ostracism make it difficult for parents or custodial guardians to seek help from natural support networks and mental health professionals.

Tibesar (1986) notes that the distinctive nature of AIDS—terminal and transmitted by specific, usually stigmatized behaviors—requires specialized responses. AIDS is concentrated among the young, thus robbing society's future and representing immeasurable economic and cultural losses. Hinton (1972) observed that younger persons are more prone to be anxious in terminal illness because dying at an early stage of life disrupts many hopes, plans, and expectations. Parents with AIDS worry about dependent children whom they are leaving behind. Some tend to suffer more physical discomfort than anxiety. Others experience cognitive impairment and suicide attempts, possibly the result of AIDS-related dementia, which can have profound effects on surviving orphans.

The AIDS epidemic in America was initially socially defined as a disease of marginalized groups in society, especially gay men, who are disproportionately affected. Press coverage referred to AIDS as the "gay plague." Little press coverage on AIDS occurred until the spring of 1983, when *The Journal of the American Medical Association* published an editorial suggesting that everyone was at risk, and *The New York Times* ran its first article on AIDS (Baker 1986; Panem 1987; Nelkin 1991). Additionally, the sociodemographic characteristics of persons infected with HIV tend to set AIDS apart from other chronic illnesses, provoking social and moral judgments regarding transmission behaviors.

Early in the epidemic, deaths from AIDS were seldom cause for general concern in African-American and Hispanic communities. Members of these communities were lulled into thinking that AIDS was "the gay, white commmunity's business." Reports that Africa and Haiti were the locus of origin of the disease angered many, who saw this attribution as an attempt to blame people of color for the disease. Rejection and discrimination against people with AIDS were widespread. Discrimination in medical care, housing, employment benefits, and insurance were regularly reported in the media, as were suggestions that people with AIDS be quarantined. Later, family and friends witnessed during their loved one's illness the denial of medical and dental care, the refusal of housekeeping personnel to clean hospital rooms, the refusal of schools to admit HIV-infected children, and the refusal of funeral directors to touch the bodies of people who had died of AIDS. The evidence was clear. People with AIDS were *personae non gratae* in the eyes of the general public, health care practitioners, and the government responsible for health care and social policies (Dane and Miller 1992).

It was, and remains, within this social context that children and adolescents orphaned by a parent's death from AIDS confront their grief, sadness, and confusion, and the mourning or public expression of that grief. As public perceptions of AIDS become inextricably tied to perceptions of the groups among which it is most prevalent, the stigmas of disease and death become attached to the groups themselves. AIDS has become a symbol: Reactions to AIDS are reactions to gay men, drug users, racial minorities, or outsiders in general (Herek and Glunt 1988).

AIDS, like cancer, "carries the indelible mark of our mortality" (Vastyn 1986)—a stark reminder that individuals are subject to pain, suffering, and death. Like cancer, AIDS confronts the survivors not only with the reality of a stigmatized death but also with fears about death and contagion, provoking what Schultz (1962) described as the "fundamental anxiety." When children or adolescents interact with a parent with AIDS, or hear AIDS discussed, they are reminded of their own mortality and how their day-to-day life has been and will be changed in a profoundly disturbing way. As Schultz suggests, the pragmatic objective of daily life is to construct experiences that avoid this fundamental anxiety.

Unlike people with cancer, however, people with AIDS are often perceived as placing others at risk for their disease (Singer et al. 1987). Also, people with HIV/AIDS often are blamed for causing their condition through risky behavior. In face-to-face encounters, the symptoms of AIDS-related illnesses, such as extreme weight loss and skin conditions, are frequently visible to others, sometimes disfiguring, and likely to disrupt a parent's social interactions. These concerns may jeopardize the family's willingness to provide care and are likely to strain a relationship. Fear of stigma may be increased by the family's knowledge that they will retain the stigma even after the death.

In order to avoid dealing publicly with the cause of death and its possible implications, surviving family members or custodial guardians may decide not to talk about the deceased parent or may circumvent traditional mourning rituals. Accurate information helps the youngster to accommodate to the reality of loss. Bowlby (1980) avers that incomplete or biased accounts of the mode of death can be detrimental to the course of grieving. Lack of information about parental death from AIDS supports the denial mechanism, which, if operative for longer than the typical period of shock, impedes bereavement. Inaccurate information, reinforced by preventing the child or adolescent from attending the funeral or failing to acknowledge the anniversary of the parent's death, enhances the tendency to disbelieve that the death actually occurred (Dunne et al. 1987).

Survivors who have a fear of sharing their grief, which is compounded when they confront multiple stressors such as illness, violence, death, or abandonment, are more likely to develop physical and psychological disorders than those who are experiencing stress from a single source (Brown and Harris 1978). Orphans of the HIV epidemic who are subjected to multiple stressors are more likely to be at risk for psychological and physical problems as the number of stressors increases. It is not unusual for families in which an AIDS death has occurred to have undergone multiple stressors before and after the death.

Many African-American and Hispanic children and adolescents live in inner cities where they daily confront the negative attitudes of the larger community. Economic resources and services are limited, and crime and violence daily threaten their lives. It takes very little imagination to visualize the social and physical environments that constantly wreak havoc on personality development, self-esteem, and a sense of personal control. For children and adolescents of color, a family member's death from AIDS intensifies their feelings of oppression and fears of being shunned by others.

Only when professionals and lay people understand the different responses to the problem among various cultures and ethnic groups will they effectively provide an empathic, caring community where children and adolescent survivors can feel safe to discuss their personal fears and openly grieve.

RELATIONSHIP TO THE DECEASED

Living in the aftermath of death from AIDS is often more painful for children and adolescents than the death itself. Some experience interminable grief and others feel anger, despair, and guilt. The questions that surround the long-term effects of parental death from AIDS bear directly upon issues that concern the general nature of parent-child relationships and offer important perspectives with regard to the relationship of early trauma and later mental illness, as well as the nature of mourning, early loss, and attachment.

Family interactions and patterns fashion the child's personality. Though the composition and style of the family vary according to class, culture, and geographic differences, its function—socialization of its young—remains the same. According to psychoanalytic theory, the family's cultural task is accomplished through a series of complex object-relations and object-representations established in early childhood and is crystallized by the outcomes of normal oedipal struggles between parents and child (Blanck and Blanck 1974; Neubauer 1960). It follows, then, that alteration in a family structure, which occurs when a parent dies of AIDS, will resound and reverberate throughout development.

While numerous factors can play a role in determining children's or adolescents' reaction to loss, the relationship of the survivor to the deceased parent and the availability of an alternate family member are important. In contrast to the early theories that strongly suggested that loss and separation in childhood (especially from the mother) were invariably pathogenic, current research stresses the importance of context and individual styles of coping in determining the effects of loss (Wolkind and Rutter 1985).

It has been suggested that mourning may not be a single process, but may entail multiple processes. Regarding the nature of grief, multiple inner representations of the lost object can be applied to children who lose a parent to AIDS. These multiple representations of the dead parent exist, and in a state of grief they are dealt with separately by the bereaved child. It is thought that each unit of representation may be related to certain biologic responses, like some memories cause one to smile or blush.

The idea of multiple inner representations has been in the clinical literature on parental death since Orbach (1988) demonstrated the complexity of parental grief in his article "The Multiple Meanings of the Loss of a Child." This notion also applies to each of the inner representations of the dead parent, which must be resolved. The resolution varies in complexity with the ambivalence in the attachment between the child and parent. Those with more inner representations which are of the less-than-good self or are extensions of attachments to negative memories of a mother who was a drug abuser, emotionally unsupportive, or unavailable in the child's and adololescent's history would produce a more difficult-to-resolve grief.

A relationship so central to the self as that between child and parent does not end with the death of the parent. Attachment theory confirms the importance of human relationships and their consequences for individual development.

Beginning in infancy, with the bond between the child and parent figure, attachments are essential to feelings of safety and security, providing care and protection during times of stress. The manner in which parents meet their child's basic strivings for attachment is an important determinant of future mental health.

When parent figures are available and responsive to their child's "attachment behaviors" for proximity and support, the child learns that others are reliable and that the self is worthy of being loved and receiving attention from others. The persistence of this sense of relationship with others is explained in terms of inner "working models" (Bowlby 1988, 129), which are mental representations that the individual builds and continually modifies through ongoing experiences. Inner-city orphans of the HIV epidemic have not always experienced the reliability that Bowlby outlines. Severe family discord, long-term stress, and trauma are likely to be the norm.

Adolescent attachment can be described as a continuation of the early mother-child bond that has become modified over time and directed toward others. Like early attachments on which they are patterned, adult bonds form slowly, with proximity and interaction, and dissolve gradually as ties weaken and undergo change (Weiss 1975; Ainsworth 1979). The capacity to resist giving up or easily replacing attachments is based on the disposition to preserve and recover bonds if they were in jeopardy. The death of a parent, which represents the loss of a close attachment, sets the process of grief and mourning in motion combined with the difficult normative demands of adolescence. Normal adolescent development calls for a set of tasks that Fleming and Adolph (1986) have described as emotional separation from parents; achievement of competency, mastery, or control; and development of intimacy versus commitment. The conflicts inherent in these tasks are separation versus reunion or abandonment versus safety, independence versus dependence, and closeness versus distance. These developmental tasks echo ambivalence, which both normally developing and adolescent mourners face with a need to achieve some separation and distance. For adolescents in particular, it is helpful to question links between their potential suicidal behavior and parental death. Ambivalence and depression are familiar features of all suicides but appear to be highly increased in suicidal adolescents.

Working within a psychoanalytic framework, Lindemann (1944) conceived of anticipatory grief as grief work performed in anticipation of the death of a love object entailing "emancipation from the bondage to the deceased, readjustment to the environment in which the deceased is missing, and the formation of new relationships" (p. 143). The notion that anticipatory grief, as a kind of rehearsal or preparation for the death of a parent, may mitigate the stress of bereavement and thus confer an adaptive advantage on the child/adolescent is intuitively appealing. While anticipatory grief may have adaptive value, no empirical research has been reported on observations of bereavement outcomes for surviving children and adolescents whose parent died of AIDS.

Generally, the death of a parent, especially for young children, creates fears for their survival. The child who has lost a parent fears that the grandparent or aunt, uncle, foster care parent may also die. The child wonders, What would then happen to me? Who would take care of me?

The child's reaction to the loss is inevitably compounded by the reactions of the custodial guardian or primary caretaker, for example, a grandmother or foster parent. Surviving parents or new caregivers must cope with adversity, the stigma from an AIDS death, and possibly their own HIV infection as they continue to be supportive of the child. If surviving parents learn that they too are HIV-positive, they may transfer dependency needs from the deceased spouse to the older children, thus stifling their needs for independence. This new relationship can seriously interfere with the adolescent's social and emotional functioning.

Surviving family members may begin to use defensive tactics to ease their own anguish. Some parents may feel responsible for their children's death if they were born HIV-infected and may be unable to talk about or explain the death or their own pending death to surviving siblings. They respond with a conspiracy of silence. In many situations, surviving children and adolescents are haunted by the fear of contagion. They fear that they could die of AIDS like their parents or young siblings. Surviving grandparents or caregivers may be consumed with their own grief and have little energy left to offer comfort, understanding, and patience. This may be compounded if there was a prolonged illness prior to the death.

In a related vein, the nature of family dynamics prior to the death must be assessed. The quality of the child's relationship to the parent affects his or her success in meeting developmental challenges prior to the death and the types and fantasies that are produced subsequent to the death. In addition to suffering grief, many children and adolescents experience guilt caused by previous arguments or fights with the dead parent. Youngsters feel in some way responsible for the death because of previous bad thoughts about their dead parents. Although the impact of parental loss can be overwhelming, it is essential to provide the kind of atmosphere where children and adolescents are given support and permission to ask questions and express feelings.

CHILDREN'S AND ADOLESCENTS'
UNDERSTANDING OF DEATH

The literature contains conflicting opinions regarding the necessity of extending professional help to the bereaved child and adolescent. Some clinicians state that the negative impact of the loss of a parent in childhood on the personality of the child is unavoidable (Freud 1960) and that crisis intervention immediately after the event in no way diminishes the danger to the psychological health of the survivors (Pollack et al. 1975).

In contrast, other researchers have confirmed the need for surviving members of the extended family, teachers, and mental health professionals to be cognizant of the wide variety of possible emotional, defensive, and behavioral reactions that the child and adolescent may demonstrate in the first few months and year of mourning. The reactions will vary; there is no standard normal or uniform reaction. Every surviving child and adolescent requires a suitable explanation of the meaning of death. The difficulty in talking to the child or adolescent lies generally in the anxieties, defenses, and confusion of the adult (Kaffman et al. 1987). The ability of the guardian or significant other to express his or her grief openly and to facilitate the child's expression of grief is of decisive importance. The age and sex of the child and adolescent (see Chapters 4 and 5) and the sex of the deceased parent frame the developmental issues. As with any aspect of development, there are large individual differences in the ages at which children and adolescents reach an understanding of death. Just as we cannot protect ourselves from life, we cannot protect bereaved children and adolescents from death.

There is widespread belief that children are not concerned with death. Freud (1953) wrote in *The Interpretation of Dreams*, "The fear of death has no meaning to a child . . . children know nothing of the horrors of corruption, of freezing in the ice cold grave, of the terrors of eternal nothingness" (p. 254) and in 1926 "Nothing resembling death can ever have been experienced; or if it has, as in fainting, it has left no observable traces behind" (p. 130). During the last decades, theorists have disproved this opinion (Furman 1974; Altschul and Beiser 1984; Fleming 1974; Gardner 1983; Eth and Pynoos 1984). It is now appreciated that children are capable of a wide range of grief responses, whose expression is influenced by the child's level of development, personality, and cultural milieu.

Grief-stricken children differ in some respects from their adult counterparts. The capacity of children to sustain sadness or dysphoric affects over time increases with age and ego maturity. Because young children have a short attention span, their sadness or pain may go unnoticed. In the preverbal child, the development of body boundaries, the rudiments of self-esteem, and basic ego functions may be at risk. A death during the oedipal period may mar sexual and characterological patterns of relating to the opposite sex. The loss of an appropriate model may be felt strongly during latency. In adolescence, the death often complicates the process of separation from parents and the establishment of an appropriate ego ideal.

In summary, bereaved younger and older children and adolescents need to receive comfort and support within their grief-stricken families. Because bereaved children and adolescents are in school most of the day, ideally family members should inform teachers or school counselors of the death, thus enabling teachers better to assist with this major loss. It is not necessary to tell the cause of death. Because of the stigma associated with death from AIDS and family rights of privacy, only with the family's permission should any school personnel be informed that the parent died of AIDS. Despite the serious problems of maintaining confidentiality, school staff's understanding that absenteeism from school, poor performance, and disruptive behavior can be related to grief can empower helping professionals to provide assistance to these orphans.

Fox (1985) has suggested four tasks that can be applied to bereaved children and adolescents. These tasks are (1) to understand what is happening or has happened, (2) to grieve or express emotional responses to the present or anticipated losses, (3) to commemorate the loss through some formal or informal remembrance, and (4) to learn how to go on with one's life.

SURVIVOR SYNDROME

Children and adolescents who grow up in an environment of continuous or even intermittent stress are likely to worry about their existence. They may assume that the world is not a safe place and that parents are unreliable. When parents die, they are left alone to cope.

Psychic trauma occurs when an individual is exposed to an overwhelming event, like parental death from AIDS, where the child or adolescent feels helpless in the face of intolerable danger, anxiety, or instinctual arousal, thus prolonging grief and mourning. When a parent dies of AIDS, the process of loss starts long before the death. Clinicians should always look for the events that the child or adolescent has experienced prior to and after the death. For many children, being orphaned results in a move from home, siblings, school, and friends. This can cause mental suffering and in some situations irreversible psychological dysfunction. Frequently, older adolescents take on increasing responsibility at home, such as parenting younger siblings without available adults.

Although trauma and grief are profoundly different human experiences, a single event can precipitate both responses. While trauma is a direct injury, the stressful situations of being orphaned by AIDS create indirect injuries. Eth and Pynoos (1984) have found that traumatic anxiety is a priority concern, compromising the ego's ability to attend to the fantasies of the lost object that are an integral part of grief work. To offset his or her traumatic helplessness, the survivor must consider, if only in fantasy, alternate actions that could have prevented the parent's death. Developmental considerations are important determinants of this cognitive effort and subsequent developmental maturity may bring about revisions.

People generally report feelings of guilt over the death of a loved one, and children and adolescents are no exception. Survivor guilt may represent a conflict over the proper assignment of human accountability. Heightened feelings of guilt arise when there has been a distortion of communication, denial, evasion, or closed discussion about the parent's death. Initially, the child or adolescent may wish to avoid the discussion, but this provides only a temporary relief. Hostile wishes, fantasies, misconduct, and other specific behavior prior to the parent's death can excerbate the guilt and self-blame. The parent's death from AIDS may be viewed as the fulfillment of angry wishes, and conscious fantasies to offset the death and save the parent are likely. Gardner (1981, 82) suggests that guilt is used as "an attempt to gain some control over this calamity, for personal control is strongly implied in the idea 'It's my fault.' " In their attempt to understand the events related to AIDS, they may assume responsibility for events over which they have no control.

On the basis of interviews with mental health practitioners in a variety of practice settings, Dane and Miller (1992) compare the emotions experienced by many of the children and adolescents orphaned by AIDS to those of youngsters who witness parental homicide, rape, or suicidal behavior. Horowitz (1980) reports that all of these children have an enormously intense perceptual, affective, and physiological experience. Two major examples of persistent physiological changes are the high frequency of sleep disturbances, including night terrors and somnambulism, and startle reactions to specific perceptual reminders. Experimental evidence indicates that, in adults, unwelcome intrusive imagery and autonomic physiological reactions can persist after a disturbing event. This response is not uncommon in children who lose a parent to AIDS.

As indicated in clinical practice, some of these orphans demonstrate symptoms fulfilling the four major DMS-III criteria for post traumatic stress disorder. In this regard they resemble traumatized children who were victims of physical and sexual abuse or kidnapping.

1. *The perceived presence of a distressing, traumatic event.* Children will often describe it as so upsetting that it will never be forgotten.
2. *The reexperiencing of the occurrence.* In young children this frequently takes the form of traumatic play and dreams, as well as intrusive images or sounds.
3. *Psychic numbing or affective constriction.* Children may exhibit subdued or mute behavior, or commonly adopt an unemotional or third-person, nearly journalistic attitude toward the event.

4. *Incident-specific phenomena that were previously not present.* Children are as likely as adults to suffer from startle reactions and avoidant behavior linked to trauma-specific reminders, and they may be especially susceptible to sleep disturbances. (Frederick 1983)

In addition, the age of the orphan affects the clinical picture and course of recovery, influencing the survivor's capacity to cope with the death and to contend with traumatic anxiety (Eth and Pynoos 1984).

Although the special vulnerability of these youngsters should be emphasized, none should be considered ill, disturbed, or exceptional. Such a stigma is likely to hinder children and adolescents in their efforts to cope and build a new positive identity for themselves. Many orphaned children and adolescents face these enormous stresses with courage and resiliency; they recover from parental loss and anticipate the future with enthusiasm and vitality. Forming new relationships, starting new families, exerting energy in school, and forming play and peer groups are ways of rebuilding their lives after their parent's death. They can accomplish these things while grieving the loss within the context of a familial or therapeutic support system.

SOCIAL SUPPORTS

There are growing awareness of and extensive literature (Lopata 1979; Raphael 1983; Vachon et al. 1980) on the idea that the bereavement process is facilitated when individuals can turn to their families, friends, and other community resources for assistance, emotional support, and empathy. Kinship in our society legitimizes grief. Reported observations of parents, teachers, mental health professionals, funeral directors, and children and adolescents clearly indicate that an AIDS death characteristically produces isolation, self-blame, and disengagement for many survivors. Since inner-city families, as well as those in urban and rural areas, risk rejection when they disclose the cause of death of their loved one, they often choose to keep it secret. In doing so, they may receive some temporary support, but the deception eventually takes its emotional toll in fear of discovery and possibly in guilt over the cover-up. The stress generated by the conspiracy of silence creates an increased isolation from social support networks and other important community resources. This "disenfranchising death" (Doka 1989) creates isolated survivors who grieve alone.

Children and adolescents are less vulnerable to surrounding pressures if they receive consistent support from family and significant others. When this social support is absent, survivors adapt by using defense mechanisms to confront the stress and divert their attention. In spite of the threat and negative consequences of being orphaned when a parent dies of AIDS, the cohesiveness and security gained from familial and extended supports allow expression of interpersonal distress and give the youngster a security net.

CONCLUSION

Since AIDS deaths increase isolation and strain important supportive relationships, multiple family treatment groups may offer opportunities for orphans and their caregivers to face issues that are taboo and provide a safe environment to communicate and work through unresolved grief feelings and enhance self-esteem.

Rather than protecting the youngster from potentially negative consequences of delayed, restrained, or unresolved grief, Excell (1991) suggests the following:

1. To allow for an open, honest, and nonjudgmental environment where questions may be asked by the child or adolescent and feelings may be discussed without fear.
2. To understand the experiences that the child or adolescent had with death and how he or she interpets these experiences.
3. To provide correct and factual information for any misperceptions the child or adolescent may have concerning death.
4. To identify a model or overview for the many feelings involved in the process of mourning.
5. To provide alternatives for the child or adolescent in saying good-bye to his or her parent (pp. 87–88).

For most African-Americans and Latinos, the religious element in the support system is significant. For those families without an organized religion as a base for that support, key persons during and after the death can fulfill this role. Postdeath activities, such as the funeral or memorial service, provide other forms of support. The opportunity to say good-bye is important, and allowing children to decide whether they wish to attend the mourning ceremonies is empowering. Not all children surviving a parent's death need a funeral to resolve their grief. But as other elements in the support system are eroded and modified by societal disdain, the funeral rituals can bring together the orphan's family, school, and recreational communities and provide an atmosphere in which to share grief and memories of the parent. Concealment or denial of pain and grief may confuse children, depending on their cognitive control of the phenomenon of death. This creates a barrier between them and the adult world, adding a second loss to the one already sustained. Although open communication is important, clinicians need to be attentive to the deleterious consequences of disclosure and the ramifications of an AIDS death.

It is essential that the family be helped to convey a clear message about the death and its related stigma. They should also be encouraged to seek individual or family counseling and to join a support group. Support groups fill an important void for bereaved orphans during a highly traumatic period of their lives. Over time, youngsters' ability to describe their grief experiences, combined with the clear message that "you will be able to enjoy life again," does much to alleviate the pain, stigma, and fears.

Grollman (1976) offers three major points, which can be applied to children and adolescents orphaned by AIDS. The first is understanding that they need to be included rather than excluded and that what is mentionable is manageable. When children are excluded, their reliance on imagination can make things a thousand times worse.

Second is providing a role model for children and adolescents. Let them know that when someone we love dies, we grieve. When they see a healthy response to loss, it is not only of value to them in the present, but also in the future when they experience other losses.

The third point is extremely important. A child's and an adolescent's personal boundaries must be respected. They may choose to react in one way or another. Forcing them into any specific reaction is as unhealthy to emotional and mental health as excluding them from any participation. Discussing the range of reactions with the custodial guardian is the responsibility of the mental health professional. The final decision belongs to the youngster.

REFERENCES

Ainsworth, D. 1979. *Cultural Cross Fire*. New York: Human Behavior Press.

Altschul, S. and H. Beiser. 1984. "The Effects of Early Parent Loss on Future Parenthood." In *Parenthood: A Psychodynamic Perspective*, eds. R. S. Cohen, B. J. Cohler, and S. H. Weissman, 173–182. New York: Guilford Press.

Baker, A. J. 1986. "The Portrayal of AIDS in the Media: An Analysis of Articles in the *New York Times*." In *The Social Dimension of AIDS*, eds. D. A. Feldman and T. M. Johnson, 179–194. New York: Praeger.

Becker, E. 1973. *The Denial of Death*. New York: Free Press.

Blanck, G. and R. Blanck. 1974. *Ego Psychology: Theory and Practice*. New York: Columbia University Press.

Bowlby, J. 1988. "Developmental Psychiatry Comes of Age." *American Journal of Psychiatry* 145:1–10.

———. 1951. *Maternal Care and Mental Health*. World Health Organization, Monograph No. 2.

———. 1980. *Attachment and Loss, Vol. 3. Loss: Sadness and Depression*. New York: Basic Books.

Bowlby, J. and E. M. Parkes. 1979. "Separation and Loss Within the Family." In *The Child in his Family*, eds. E. J. Anthony and C. Koupernik. New York: John Wiley and Sons.

Bowling, A. and A. Cartwright. 1982. *Life After a Death: A Study of the Elderly Widowed*. New York: Tavistock.

Brown, G. W. and T. Harris. 1978. *Social Origins of Depression*. New York: Free Press.

Christ, G. H. and L. S. Wiener. 1985. "Psychosocial Issues in AIDS." In *AIDS Etiology Diagnosis Treatment and Prevention*, eds. V. T. DeVita, Jr., S. Hellman, and S. Rosenberg, 275–297. Philadelphia: J. B. Lippincott.

Dane, B. O. 1990. "AIDS and Dying: The Teaching Challenge. *Journal of Teaching in Social Work* 4:85–100.

Dane, B. O. and S. O. Miller. 1992. *AIDS: Intervening with Hidden Grievers*. Westport, CT: Auburn House.

Danforth, L. M. 1982. *The Death Rituals of Rural Greece*. Princeton, NJ: Princeton University Press.

Dial, A. L. 1978. "Death and Life of Native Americans." *The Indian Historian* 11:32–37.

Doka, K. J. 1987. "Silent Sorrow: Grief and the Loss of Significant Others." *Death Studies* 11:455–469.

———. 1989. *Disenfranchised Grief: Recognizing Hidden Sorrow*. Lexington, MA: Lexington Books.

Dracopoulou, S., and S. Doxiadis. 1988. "In Greece, Lament for the Dead, Denial for the Dying." *The Hastings Center Report* 18(4): 15–16. Supplement.

Dunne, E., J. McIntosh, and M. K. Dunne, eds. 1987. *Suicide and Its Aftermath: Understanding and Counseling the Survivors*. New York: W. W. Norton.

Eth, S. and R. Pynoos. 1984. *Post-Traumatic Stress Disorder in Children*. Washington, DC: American Psychiatric Press.

Excell, S. 1991. "A Child's Perception of Death." In *Children and Death*, eds. D. Papadatau and C. Papadatos. New York: Hemisphere Publishing.

Fleming, J. 1974. "The Problem of Diagnosis in Parent Loss Cases." *Contemporary Psychoanalysis* 10:439–451.

Fleming, S. and R. Adolph. 1986. "Helping Bereaved Adolescents: Needs and Responses." In *Adolescence and Death,* eds. C. Carr and J. McNeil, 97–118. New York: Praeger Press.

Forstein, M. 1984. "AIDS Anxiety in the 'Worried Well.'" In *Psychiatric Aspects of Acquired Immune Deficiency Syndrome*, eds. S. E. Nichols and D. G. Ostrow. Washington, DC: American Psychiatric Press.

Fox, S. S. 1984/1985. "Children's Anniversary Reactions to the Death of a Family Member." *Omega* 150.

Frederick, J. E. 1983. "The Biochemistry of Bereavement: Possible Basis for Chemotherapy?" *Omega* 13:295–303.

Freud, S. 1953. *Interpretation of Dreams*. Chapter 5, footnote 1909, 1900. In *The Standard Edition of the Complete Psychological Works of Sigmund Freud*, ed. J. Strachey, 4. London: Hogarth Press.

———. 1960. "Discussion of Dr. Bowlby's Paper." *Psychoanalytic Study of the Child* 15:53.

———. 1968. "Thoughts for the Times on War and Death." In *Civilisation, War and Death: Sigmund Freud*, ed. J. Rickman, 1–25. London: Hogarth Press.

Furman, E. 1974. *A Child's Parent Dies: Studies in Childhood Bereavement*. New Haven, CT: Yale University Press.

Gardner, R. A. 1981. "Death of a Parent." In *Basic Handbook of Child Psychiatry*, ed.
J. D. Noshpitz, 4. New York: Basic Books.

Geis, S. B., R. L. Fuller, and J. Rush. 1986. "Lovers of AIDS Victims: Psychosocial
Stresses and Counseling Needs." *Death Studies* 10:43–53.

Glick, I. O., R. Weiss, and C. M. Parkes. 1974. *The First Year of Bereavement*. New
York: John Wiley and Sons.

Goffman, E. 1963. *Stigma: Notes on the Management of Spoiled Identity*. Englewood
Cliffs, NJ: Prentice Hall.

Grollman, E. A. 1976. *Talking About Death: A Dialogue Between Parent and Child*.
Boston: Beacon Press.

Herek, G. M. and E. K. Glunt. 1988. "An Epidemic of Stigma: Public Reactions to
AIDS." *American Psychologist* 43:886–891.

Hinton, J. 1972. *Dying*. Baltimore: Penguin Books.

Hoagland, J. 1984. "Bereavement and Personal Constructs: Old Theories and New
Concepts." *Death Education* 2:175–193.

Holmes, T. H. and R. H. Rahe. 1967. "The Social Readjustment Rating Scale."
Journal of Psychosomatic Research 11:213–218.

Horowitz, M. J. and N. Kaltreider. 1980. "Brief Treatment of Post Traumatic Stress
Disorders." *New Directions for Mental Health Services* 6:67–79.

Jones, E. E., A. Farina, and A. H. Hastorf. 1984. *Social Stigma: The Psychology of
Marked Relationships*. New York: Freeman.

Kaffman, M., E. Elizur, and L. Gluckson. 1987. "Bereavement Reactions in Children: Therapeutic Implications." *Israel Journal of Psychiatry Science* 24:1–2,
65–76.

Kubler-Ross, E. 1969. *On Death and Dying*. New York: Macmillan.

Lifton, R. 1979. *The Broken Connection*. New York: Simon and Schuster.

Lindemann, E. 1944. "The Symptomatology and Management of Acute Grief."
American Journal of Psychiatry 101:141–148.

Lopata, H. Z. 1979. *Women as Widows*. New York: Elsevier North Holland.

Marshall, V. W. 1980. *Last Chapters: The Sociology of Aging and Dying*. Monterey,
CA: Brooks/Cole.

Meissner, W. 1988. "Impending Nuclear Disaster: Psychoanalytic Perspectives." In
Psychoanalysis and the Nuclear Threat, eds. H. Levine, D. Jackobs, and L.
Rubins, 89–110. Hillsdale, NJ: Analytic Press.

Morin, S. F., K. A. Charles, and A. K. Malyon. 1984. "The Psychological Impact of
AIDS on Gay Men." *American Psychologist* 39:1288–1293.

Nelkin, D. 1991. "AIDS and the News Media." *Milbank Quarterly* 69:293–307.

Neubauer, P. B. 1960. "The One-Parent Child and his Oedipal Development."
Psychoanalytic Study of the Child 15:286–309.

Orbach, I. 1988. *Children Who Don't Want to Live*. San Francisco: Jossey-Bass.

Palombo, J. 1981. "Parent Loss and Childhood Bereavement: Some Theoretical
Considerations." *Clinical Social Work Journal* 9:3–33.

Panem, S. 1987. *The AIDS Bureaucracy*. Cambridge, MA: Harvard University Press.

Parkes, C. M., and R. S. Weiss. 1972. "Components of the Reaction to Loss of a
Limb, Spouse or Home." *Journal of Psychosomatic Research* 16:343–349.

———. 1983. *Recovery from Bereavement*. New York: Basic Books.

Peppers, L., and R. Knapp. 1980. *Motherhood and Mourning*. New York: Praeger.

Petropoulos, D. 1959. *Ellinika Dimotika Tragoudia*. Athens, Greece: Zaharopoulos.

Pollack, P., D. Egan, R. Vandervergh, and V. Williams. 1975. "Prevention in Mental Health: A Controlled Study." *American Journal of Psychiatry* 132:146–149.

Raphael, B. 1983. *The Anatomy of Bereavement*. New York: London: Hutchinson, Basic Books.

Rickman, J. 1968. *Civilisation, War and Death: Sigmund Freud*. London: Hogarth Press.

Rosenblatt, P. C., R. P. Walsh, and D. A. Jackson. 1976. *Grief and Mourning in Cross-Cultural Perspective*. New York: HRAF Press.

Rudestam, K. E. 1977. "Physical and Psychological Response to Suicide in the Family." *Journal of Consulting and Clinical Psychology* 45:167–170.

Sanders, C. H. 1979/1980. "A Comparison of Adult Bereavement in the Death of a Spouse, Child and Parent." *Omega* 10:303–322.

Schultz, A. 1962. "Multiple Realities." In *Collected Papers, Vol. 1: The Problem of Social Reality*, ed. M. Natanson, 207–259. The Hague: Nijhoff.

Segal, H. 1988. "Silence is the Real Crime." In *Psychoanalysis and the Nuclear Threat*, eds. H. Levin, D. Jacobs, and L. Rubin, 35–58. Hillsdale, NJ: Analytic Press.

Silko, L.M. 1974. "The Man to Send Rain Clouds" In *The Man to Send Rain Clouds: Contemporary Stories by American Indians*." In K. Rosen Ed. New York: Viking Press, pp. 3–8.

Simos, B. G. 1979. *A Time to Grieve: Loss as a Universal Human Experience*. Milwaukee: Family Service America.

Singer, E., T. F. Rogers, and M. Cocoran. 1987. "The Polls, a Report: AIDS." *Public Opinion Quarterly* 51:580–595.

Tibesar, L. 1986. "Pastoral Care: Helping Patients on an Inward Journey." *Health Progress* 67:41–47.

Vachon, M.L.S., A. R. Sheldon, W. J. Lancee, W.A.L. Lyall, J. Rogers, and S.J.J. Freeman. 1980. "A Controlled Study of Self-Help Intervention for Widows." *American Journal of Psychiatry* 137:1380–1384.

Vastyn, E. 1986. "Spiritual Aspects of the Care of Cancer Patients." *Cancer Journal for Clinicians* 36:110–114.

Viorst, J. 1986. *Necessary Losses*. New York: Simon and Schuster.

Volkan, V.D. 1972. "The Linking of Objects of Pathological Mourners." *Archives of General Psychiatry* 27:215–221.

Weiss, R. S. 1975. *Marital Separation*. New York: Basic Books.

Wolkind, S., and M. Rutter. 1985. "Separation Loss and Family Relationships." In *Child and Adolescent Psychiatry: Modern Approaches*, eds. Rutter and Hersov. London: Blackwell Scientific.

3

Suffer the Little Children: The Child and Spirituality in the AIDS Crisis

Kenneth J. Doka

INTRODUCTION

When a little girl holds a dead bird in her hands and plaintively asks "Why?" she is asking a profoundly spiritual question. A meaningful answer will have little to do with stopped hearts, the lack of respiration, or the cessation of nerve impulses. The question transcends those biophysical concerns. It asks no less than the meaning of life.

Death is a spiritual crisis. It demands answers beyond the realm of immediate experiences. Throughout the years, social work and psychological literature have recognized that death, especially the death of a parent, is a psychological and social crisis for the child. Yet, the spiritual nature of the crisis has all but been ignored.

This chapter seeks to address that issue. Specifically it speaks to two points. First, given the nature of a parental death from AIDS, it asks how religion and spiritual beliefs and rituals can complicate or facilitate the bereavement process. Second, it addresses the ways that caregivers can understand, evaluate and energize a child's belief system and faith community in order to ameliorate his or her grief. To consider those issues, it is first necessary both to explore the development of a child's spirituality and to review the spiritual dimensions of AIDS.

Even before that, however, it is important to state two initial assumptions. First, this chapter makes a distinction between religion and spirituality. The concept of spirituality is used in the broadest possible context; it refers to anything transcendental, that is, anything beyond the material body. Religion, ethics, supernatural beliefs, love, and nonmaterialistic philosophies are all dimensions of spirituality. Religion is more narrowly defined as a formal, theistic belief system. To put it simply, a child may be defined religiously as a Roman Catholic, Muslim, or Baptist. That child's spirituality, although it may include some of the beliefs indicated by formal and informal religious training, may also include other transcendental beliefs such as beliefs in voodoo, ghosts, or spells. This reminds caregivers of an important point. Spirituality is highly individual and only partially defined by the religious belief system. Furthermore, many religious systems have a variety of interpretations of their own traditions. Thus simply trying to define anyone's spirituality, child or adult, by simply referring to religious affiliation is clearly inadequate.

Second, spirituality is deeply linked to one's culture. The Roman Catholicism of Puerto Rican Americans is far different from that of their Haitian or Irish counterparts. The Islam practiced by an African-American may be far different from that of an Iranian-American. Even the Baptist faith of an African-American migrant from the South may be different from a more urbanized, northern black. Each child's spirituality has to be understood within its own cultural context.

THE CHILD'S SPIRITUAL DEVELOPMENT

The study of a child's spiritual development has been an empirical lacuna. Most of the scant research available has taken a developmental perspective, heavily influenced by Piagetian models. Most developmentalists have tended to emphasize that young children have not developed the abilities of abstract thought necessary to embrace religion. For example, Nye and Carlson (1984) emphasize that children under 10 or 11 years of age do not have the cognitive capabilities demanded for an adequate notion of God. Similarly, Lonetto (1980) notes that children under 12 years of age think too concretely to develop profound spiritual insights.

Developmental perspectives generally have been criticized for emphasizing what children are incapable of doing without adequately stressing what they are trying to do. Coles (1990), in his extensive study of spirituality and its development in children, offers that latter alternative. To Coles children are pilgrims on a journey in which they are trying to make sense of their world. Coles emphasizes that children incorporate many of the beliefs that they are exposed to even when they are very young.

In some homes where religion is more explicitly and constantly evoked—rituals practiced, mandates and rules enforced—spiritual values become for children part and parcel of the emotional life they struggle to consolidate for themselves. (1990, 127)

Coles further describes how religious and biblical stories, which children may understand differently at different ages, become models and sources of inspiration. He also discusses how spirituality is often related to the broad religious themes such as Islamic surrender to the power of Allah, Christian salvation, and Jewish righteousness. This struggle to create meaning is often intense when children are confronted with suffering, illness, and death.

Under such circumstances, psychological themes connect almost imperceptibly, but quite vividly, at moments with a spiritual inwardness (Coles 1990, 101). And again, it seems that religious backgrounds provide distinct alternatives for understanding and interpreting these events (Candy-Gibbs et al. 1985).

A child's development will affect the ways he or she understands and expresses spirituality. This is particularly important when dealing with orphans of the HIV epidemic, some of whom, given their pre- and postnatal environments, may have developmental deficits. But the question is not at what age or developmental level children can understand spiritual concepts. Rather the question should be, How does the child, at this age and developmental level, understand and express his or her spirituality?

SPIRITUALITY AND THE CRISIS OF AIDS

Any death, especially the death of a parent, raises spiritual questions for the child. Questions such as "Why did this happen?", "Why did it happen to me?", and "Why did he, she, or they have to die?" are inherently spiritual. Even questions such as "What will happen to me?" and "Who will take care of me?" have spiritual dimensions.

While any death raises profound questions of meaning, AIDS-related deaths may be particularly problematic. First, the tremendous fear and stigma attached to AIDS can generate a context where children find it difficult to seek support either from peers or from adults. Many children learn very early that their parent's disease is shrouded in secrecy. They may personally experience the stigma of AIDS-related illness, as they are teased by classmates or ostracized by peers and other parents. Because AIDS engenders such dread, survivors of AIDS-related deaths are often reluctant or ashamed to share their secret with others. And that can make the quest to find meaning even more difficult.

To complicate the issue further, for many, AIDS has profound moral implications. Kowaleski (1990) notes that there are three different religious constructions of the AIDS crisis. In one, a common perspective in more fundamentalist and conservative faiths, AIDS is a divine punishment for moral failures of homosexuality and drug abuse. In this perspective, while some may be innocent victims, most persons with AIDS are responsible for their affliction and deserve their fate. A second construction, evident in many churches such as the Roman Catholic Church, also see AIDS as a consequence of moral failure. However, the church emphasizes loving the sinner even while condemning the sin. In this perspective, while many persons with AIDS may be responsible for their own condition, they deserve compassion and help. Kowaleski (1990) labels a third construction "embracing the exile." In this perspective, there is no notion of AIDS as a punishment for moral failure. Rather, the limited response of organized religion is seen as its moral failure. This perspective may be shared by more liberal churches. The point is that many children may be affiliated with church bodies that offer very mixed or negative images of persons with AIDS. These images may complicate the child's own spiritual constructions.

A second complicating factor is the chaotic nature of the lives of many orphans of the epidemic. Many face the constant difficulties of living with poverty and deprivation. Many are the children of drug users. In some cases both parents may have engaged in drug use or other antisocial behaviors. The child may have been in and out of drug programs or prisons. At times the child's own care may have been neglected. The child may have lived, at times, with relatives or family friends in an informal system of foster care. The child may have been in the formal foster care system living in perhaps a number of foster homes, including kinship homes.

HIV illness itself can also be chaotic. It is characterized by uncertainty and unpredictability. In lower income homes, illness can be especially difficult to manage. Again, depending upon available support and the course of the illness, the child's needs—psychological, social, and spiritual—may be ignored. And again, during the course of the illness, if not prior to it, they may find themselves living with a variety of caregivers.

This, too, complicates the spiritual struggle. Some children, given their environment, may experience developmental or behavioral problems. They may find it difficult to trust or to bond with adults. They may experience a lack of consistency even in facing their own spiritual struggles.

They may have to struggle with the issue of multiple loss. Many of these children may have lost both parents—through AIDS, abandonment, inability to care for them, or for other reasons. They may have experienced the loss of other family members. They may have been separated from other caregivers such as foster parents. The very nature of foster care placement may involve separations from siblings, friends, neighbors, and classmates. It is hard enough to struggle with spiritual questions of meaning when one has experienced a single loss; it is even more difficult with multiple losses.

RELIGION AND SPIRITUALITY: IMPLICATIONS FOR CAREGIVERS

Religion and spirituality can complicate or facilitate a child's response to illness, loss, and death. In order to understand the ways that the child's spirituality affects his or her response to loss, caregivers have to explore the child's beliefs, understand the rituals the child has participated in or could find meaningful, and assess whether or not the child might be connected to a supportive faith community.

Understanding the Spiritual Framework

The first thing the caregiver needs to do is to understand the child's spiritual framework. Once trust and rapport have been established, this can best be accomplished by open-ended questions. What happens to a person when he or she dies? Do you attend church or Sunday school? These simple and direct questions can start conversations about spirituality at an appropriate level.

If the child is wearing any religious symbols such as a cross, crescent, or star, these too can be appropriate topics with which to begin. Where did you get such a beautiful cross? What does it mean to you? Stories and play can also be effective ways to broach conversation about spirituality. For example, a deeply spiritual conversation with one young 7-year-old boy began when I noticed a Sunday school pin on his shirt. We then talked about some recent lessons. The child drew pictures and told the Old Testament story of Joseph. When I asked him about the meaning of the story, he stated that it showed that God cared about people even when they were in strange places away from their families.

The child's spiritual framework can include many types of beliefs that do not necessarily come from religion but from other sources. One child, for example, told me that her mother was now a ghost. To this 10-year-old girl, very good people become angels when they die. Bad people become skeletons. People in the middle, like her mother, a former IV drug user, become ghosts. In this state they have a final opportunity to be good or bad ghosts before their fate was settled.

A few comments about this child's beliefs: First, many of them are clearly derived from popular cultural images; witness the success of the movie *Ghost*, and others with similar themes. Second, her belief provides a structure to explore and resolve her strongly ambivalent feelings toward her mother. Finally, her beliefs have the potential to provide considerable comfort.

Not all spiritual frameworks are so comforting. Many beliefs may be quite troubling. Understanding and exploring these beliefs can allow the child the opportunity to develop different understandings.

Caregivers first need to understand the child's spiritual framework. This can be accomplished in a number of ways, using conversations, stories, art, music, or any other approaches in ways appropriate to the child's developmental level. Caregivers should be patient in their approach. Children may be unsure and confused about the varieties of spiritual images they hold, and reluctant to share them with adults. And, of course, counselors should be respectful. Sources for spiritual information can be diverse, including parents, other adults, peers, formal and informal religious instruction, and media—all filtered through the child's own perception. Gently sorting out these beliefs and seeing how they connect and influence grieving are time-consuming processes. Condescending demeanor, judgmental attitudes, or dismissal of beliefs can terminate this process at any point.

Once the child's spiritual framework is understood, caregivers can utilize that framework in facilitating grief. For example, if a child is feeling guilty, perhaps he or she can find comfort in spiritual beliefs. One young Puerto Rican child, fresh from his First Communion, a major family event, was able to confess his anger and jealousy at a younger brother whose own HIV illness absorbed considerable family attention. The absolution and encouragement of a sympathetic family priest did much to resolve his feelings.

Beliefs may also allow the child to maintain a therapeutic attachment to the deceased parent. In recent years concepts of grief have begun to emphasize that for many grievers, maintaining an attachment to the deceased may be very therapeutic (Doka 1993; Hogan 1993; Silverman et al. 1992). For children and adolescents, beliefs about an afterlife often provide ways to maintain that attachment. For example, Silverman, Nickman, and Worden's (1992) study of children experiencing parental loss found that many of the children were comforted by their beliefs that their parents were in heaven and were able to remain involved, at some level, in their lives. Hogan (1993), in her study of bereaved adolescent siblings, reported similar results.

Effectively Utilizing Religious and Spiritual Rituals

One of the most powerful manifestations of spirituality lies in rituals. At their best, rituals can be highly therapeutic. They can provide psychological comfort, social support, and spiritual meaning.

For many children the power of therapeutic rituals is untapped. The reasons for this are twofold. In some cases, the child simply does not have the opportunity to attend or participate in rituals, perhaps because the child is not living with the parent at this point or because caregivers wish to protect the child from what is perceived to be a troubling or problematic event. In other cases, the child is unprepared for the ritual. The ritual then is meaningless or frightening.

One of the most significant rituals is, of course, the funeral. Persons may have considerable feeling about whether children should attend funerals. My own perspective is that if the child is able to sit through a gathering, the child should have the right to choose whether or not to attend. For a child to choose appropriately, he or she will need information and alternatives. For the ritual to be meaningful, the child will need support and a meaningful role.

In preparing a child to make a decision on whether or not to attend a funeral, caregivers can begin by explaining what the funeral is and what is likely to occur. They can describe its purpose, the physical setting, the ways in which people are expected to behave, and the range of reactions that the child may observe. This will involve understanding the funeral's cultural and religious context. Children should be told that people may sob or cry because they miss the person or they may even laugh as they remember funny or happy stories about the person who died. Caregivers can assure the child that any decision that the child makes is appropriate and will be understood. Patiently answer any questions.

If the child is really going to decide, the child will need viable alternatives. If a younger child's only alternative is to stay home in an empty house, it is not a true choice. If possible, arrangements should be made for the child to stay with a sympathetic and trusted adult.

Alternatives should be reasonable. One child was given an alternative of going to her father's funeral or going on a very special outing to a place she had long wanted to see. Years later, she still felt guilty about her choice of the trip.

Options and alternatives also mean participating in ways that are comfortable. There are many decisions regarding the child's participation in a funeral ritual: whether he or she will attend a service, be present at a viewing, go up to the casket, or touch the deceased. Even if the child does not choose to attend, there may be other alternatives that can give the child a meaningful sense of participation, for example, writing a note that is included in the casket.

It is also critical that the child have support. Each child should have a supportive adult whose main function is to maintain the child's psychological comfort. This person can answer questions, provide nurturing, and, if necessary, remove the child.

The child should also have an opportunity to participate and personalize the ritual. Writing a note, placing a gift in the casket, even handing out flowers at the grave site may allow the child a sense of therapeutic empowerment.

Significant rituals do not always have to be centered around the funeral. Other public rituals such as commemorative masses or memorial services, or even private rituals such as lighting candles or prayer, may also be therapeutic. One woman whose gay brother died of AIDS found it very meaningful that her son, the deceased's nephew, took his late uncle's name as a middle name when he was confirmed.

Rituals do not have to be overtly religious. In one case an 8-year old child felt guilty that he had never told his father he loved him. He designed a ritual to bring closure. He dedicated flowers in his church "in loving memory of his father." He then placed those flowers on the grave, telling his father that he loved him.

Energizing the Faith and Faith Community

Finally, caregivers can assist the child by helping to energize the child's faith and faith community. A major thesis of this chapter has been that the beliefs and rituals of the child's spirituality, however defined, have the potential to facilitate the child's adjustment to illness, loss, and death.

Caregivers should also seek to enlist and encourage the child's faith community. Churches and temples can be significant sources of strengths. Clergy and church families can be strong support, a fact well documented in African-American communities. Caregivers should strive to build connections or reconnections that may have been initially withdrawn out of fear or shame. Regardless of the belief structure, many churches and temples can offer a warm and loving environment where children and their caregivers can be nurtured.

CONCLUSION

The death of a parent is certainly a profound psychological and social crisis for a child, especially when that parent dies from AIDS. It is also a spiritual crisis, where the child, at different points in his or her development, seeks meanings for the event. To ignore that spiritual crisis, and to fail to utilize the strengths of the child's own spiritual beliefs, rituals, and community, is, at best, less than holistic care.

To Coles the role of a supportive adult, whether a counselor, parent or other caregiver, is to recognize in the child a fellow pilgrim:

to enter that territory whose character none here ever knows. Yet how young we are when we start wondering about it all, the nature of the journey and of the final destination. (1990, 335)

Or as it was said much earlier:

Let the children come to me, and do not hinder them; for such belong to the kingdom of God. (Luke 18:16, RSV)

REFERENCES

Candy-Gibbs, Sandra, Kay Sharp, and Craig Petron. 1985. "The Effects of Age, Object, and Cultural Religious Background on Children's Conception of Death." *Omega* 15:329–46.

Coles, Robert. 1990. *The Spiritual Life of Children*. Boston: Houghton Mifflin.

Doka, Kenneth J. 1993. "The Many Roads of Resolution." Paper presented to The Association for Death Education and Counseling. Memphis, TN, April.

Hogan, Nancy. 1993. "Adolescent Responses to Sibling Bereavement." Presented to Houston Grief Center Conference. Houston, TX, March.

Kowaleski, Mark. 1990. "Religious Constructions of the AIDS Crisis." *Sociological Analysis* 51:91–96.

Lonetto, Richard. 1980. *Children's Conception of Death*. New York: Springer.

Nye, W. Chad, and Jerry Carlson. 1984. "The Development of the Concept of God in Children." *Journal of Genetic Psychology* 145:137–142.

Silverman, Phyllis, Steven Nickman, and William Worden. 1992. "Detachment Revisited: The Child's Reconstruction of the Dead Parent." *American Journal* 62:494–503.

4

Parental Loss and Latency Age Children

Karolynn Siegel
Barbara Freund

As Furman (1964) has observed, no other childhood event is as psychologically significant as the death of a parent because it deprives the child of so much opportunity to love and be loved. This chapter will focus on the nature of bereavement in latency age children (ages 6–11). Specifically, it will review what is known about mourning in young children, the significance of childhood bereavement for their later social and emotional development, and children's emotional and behavioral responses to parental death. It also includes suggestions and recommendations for facilitating children's psychosocial adjustment to the death of a parent from AIDS.

CONSEQUENCES FOR PERSONALITY AND SOCIAL-EMOTIONAL DEVELOPMENT OF THE LOSS OF A PARENT IN CHILDHOOD

The loss of a parent during childhood is perhaps the most devastating trauma a child can experience. The death results in a disorganization of family life and disruption of its unity. This may cause young children to begin to view their world as unpredictable. They can respond with a heightened sense of vulnerability, often marked by fears of recurrent tragedy. For example, they may worry that other members of their family will also die (Arthur and Kemme 1964). These fears and separation anxieties, which almost always occur when a child loses a parent, become more meaningful and profound when a parent dies of AIDS because the child may well have to confront the loss of multiple family members to the same disease. The loss of a parent in childhood can also profoundly alter children's intrapsychic world and capacity for future growth. As Sekaer (1987) has noted, children define themselves in large part through the quality of their relationships with their parents. Their evolving sense of who they are is significantly influenced by the emotional life they share with their parents.

Sekaer (1987) stresses that the younger child in particular maintains a special type of relationship with parents, which forms an essential part of the child's personality. The child very much identifies with his parents and internalizes parental images. Parental death typically represents an abrupt interruption in the process of identification and evolution of the self.

At different stages and in different ways, parents complete the child's personality until adulthood. This process, concisely described by Furman (1974), involves young children's dependency on others for fulfillment of bodily needs. They are both physically and psychologically dependent on their parents, who assist and nurture them by providing everyday sustenance. As they grow and develop, they become less dependent on their parents and more self-sufficient. Parents, however, still provide essential assistance in areas such as impulse control, inner and outer reality testing, and as models for identification. As adolescents move into adulthood, they struggle against parents and begin to form new outside relationships and important new identifications.

DEVELOPMENT AS A FACTOR IN RESPONSE TO THE LOSS

The child's developmental level, which includes the ability to understand the meaning of the death cognitively, is a crucial variable in the child's response to parental loss. Some theorists believe that prior to age 3 or 4 the concept of death is far too abstract for children's immature cognition and language development. Sekaer (1987) points out, however, that others believe that by age 2 or 3 children are able to understand the external fact of their loss and to experience the corresponding inner changes. Schaefer and Lyons (1986) explain that as children progress from age 3 to about age 6 they begin to gain some limited understanding of death, but generally do not regard death as final. They regard death as reversible and believe that the deceased may return at some future date. For these children, those who are dead are simply "less alive." Children at this age may often regard death as similar to sleep.

Schaefer and Lyons (1986) contend that young children cannot even grasp the notion of a world without their parents. Magical thinking, which provides children with imaginary special powers, is very evident at this age. In their wish to have their deceased mother or father return, children will believe a strong urge or wish is enough to bring the dead person back to life.

For example, Ben, age 8, whose mother had died of AIDS two months earlier believed that if he was able to keep his mother's plants alive, she would eventually return.

As the child gets older, the capacity for abstract thinking increases as part of normal development and maturation. Camper et al. (1991) note that significant issues to consider with latency age children are their expanding intellect, their need for academic mastery, and their increased connections to the outside world. By age 7 or 8, children have the capacity to begin to grasp the finality of death. By ages 10 and 11, the causes of death can be understood, and death is perceived as final, inevitable, and associated with the abrupt stopping of bodily activities (Camper et al. 1991; Osterweis et al. 1984).

Latency age children often appear able to accept and discuss a death on one level and yet simultaneously deny it on another level. Schaefer and Lyons (1986) explain that younger latency age children will look upon death as a taker, something violent that may come and grab them. They also often believe death is contagious. For children who have lost a parent to AIDS, this belief is often intensified because they may suffer multiple losses from the same disease. For these children in particular, the ways in which HIV is transmitted need to be explained in an age-appropriate manner to reassure them of their own bodily safety.

Older latency age children, Schaefer and Lyons (1986) note, may often experience an inner struggle around issues of morality and ethics. This too can take on special meaning for children whose parent acquired HIV through sexual transmission or drug use. Children this age may view their parent's death as a punishment for their own "bad" behavior or thoughts, leaving them feeling confused and guilty. "Most children on some level are contending with the notion that their own aggressive behaviors, misbehavior or evil thoughts had been instrumental in the death. Sometimes the child both fears and fantasizes the deceased parent will return to seek revenge upon the child" (Schaefer and Lyons 1986).

Finally, Camper et al. (1991) note that at this age, children are very interested in the biological details of what happened. A latency age child may sometimes baffle others by asking seemingly cold and scientific questions regarding a parent's death. This type of questioning, however, is often an adaptive method of coping.

Susan, age 11, whose father was within days of dying of AIDS, asked her grandmother very matter-of-factly, "Will daddy's body be cold, as soon as he dies?"

Damon, age 10, whose mother had died only a couple of weeks earlier, asked her older step-brother, "How long will it be before mommy's body looks like a skeleton?"

CAN CHILDREN MOURN? DIFFERENCES BETWEEN
CHILD AND ADULT MOURNING

According to Baker, Sedney and Gross (1992), "Children differ from adults in their cognitive abilities, their coping styles, their need for identification figures, and their dependence on adults for support. These developmental differences will affect how children approach and accomplish the tasks of grieving" (p. 114).

Children's capacity for mourning has long been a subject of debate. While most theorists agree that children react to the loss, questions have been raised regarding whether the child has the internal developmental capacity for complete "mourning" (as in adult mourning) to take place. Complete mourning is based on a psychoanalytic model that posits that full resolution of the loss cannot occur until the grieving individual detaches memories and hopes from the dead person (Sekaer 1987; Miller 1971). Osterweis, Solomon, and Green (1984) note that for children to be able to do this, they must (1) have some understanding of the concept of death, (2) be capable of forming a real attachment bond, and (3) have a mental representation of the attachment figure.

Sekaer (1987) notes that some theorists contend that young children lack the ego strength to tolerate the intense pain of mourning and therefore cannot carry out the work of mourning. Others believe the child is unable internally to let go of the parent even after death because of his inner wish and need for parental nurturance. Even those theorists who do believe children have the capacity to mourn argue against a perspective using an adult model in which the person must internally give up the deceased person. Bowlby (1980), for example, described three stages of childhood mourning. The first is a stage of protest, which is the child's attempt to deny the death. At this stage the child still believes that he can regain the dead parent by reproaching the parent for his abandonment. This is followed by pain, despair, and disorganization. Regression at this second stage is very common, as the child feels overwhelmed by the onslaught of feelings, thoughts, and memories. Finally, in the third stage, hope prevails as the child begins to reorganize his life without the lost person.

Abby, age 9, reacted to her mother's death from AIDS with unusual silence. Abby refused all attempts by her father and other close family members to talk about any feelings related to how much she missed her mother. Abby removed from her bedroom all the photographs of her mother and would leave any room in which people were discussing her mother's memory. It seemed as if Abby was trying to create an atmosphere in which she could pretend that the death in fact had not occurred.

A few months later Abby's behavior began to change. She developed sleep problems and became unusually hostile in her actions toward others, particularly her younger siblings. In addition, Abby became very emotional in all her interactions, and would cry almost incessantly.

In some ways this regressive behavior provided her father with a chance to begin to help Abby work through her intense feelings of loss and abandonment. In fact, over time Abby became more emotionally accessible in her ability to talk not only about how much she missed her mother but also how angry she was toward her mother for leaving her.

Critics of those who question whether children are capable of mourning believe it is wrong to require children to fit into a preexisting model of adult processes of mourning, and they advocate a separate model specific to the needs of children. They contend that it is not viable to use an adult model of grief and bereavement with children who are still very much in the process of cognitive and emotional development.

At least two fundamental differences between adult mourning and child mourning have been identified. First, as already stated, adults will eventually detach memories and hopes from the dead person (Schaefer and Lyons 1986; Furman 1974). In coping with a loss, Miller (1971) notes, children have a completely different goal. Children work hard both to avoid and to accept the reality of death. While acknowledging the loss of the parent in the external world, children try very hard in their inner world to maintain the relationship they have lost in their outer world.

Second, children's mourning tends to be more intermittent than that of adults. Because of children's more limited capacities to confront and manage the emotional impact of the loss, they will tend to alternate between periods of mourning and periods of not acknowledging the loss or pain. That is, they follow a kind of pattern of approach, avoidance, approach, and so on.

CHILDREN'S REACTION TO THE LOSS/WAYS OF COPING

Arthur and Kemme (1964) state, "Each child's emotional response to death will, of course, be multi-faceted and to a certain extent, peculiar to him as an individual depending, among other factors, upon his developmental level, his prior relationship to the deceased, and the manner in which the family copes with the disruption of their unity" (p. 40). However, there are a number of common reactions.

Denial clearly plays a central role in how children cope with the death of a parent. They will often try to deny the existence of a traumatic event. They may be sad and upset upon hearing the news of a death, but often this visible show of emotion lasts only a short time. Children are sometimes found playing or watching television shortly after hearing profoundly bad news. This phenomenon, or "short sadness span," in reference to the limits of a child's tolerance for confronting the pain of the loss, is one important difference in children's and adults patterns of mourning. In this behavior, it may appear that the child does not understand what has happened (Wessel 1973). In fact the child is very aware of the death. This seemingly nonchalant behavior is a way for the child to cope with intense feelings of fear and desertion. The child tries to carry on as usual in an attempt to see the world as it was before, and act as if nothing has happened.

Lionel, age 7, returned from his mother's funeral to a house full of guests visibly upset and grieving. He appeared indifferent to the circumstances and was insistent about being allowed to go over to a friend's house to watch videos.

Wessel (1973) further notes that these children may find it easier to express their sadness over someone or something less emotionally meaningful to them than the parent. Children are often found crying and feeling sad about something far less significant than their parent's death. It's not unusual, for example, to find a child crying over a sad book in which a main character has died. It is easier for the child to express grief about a fictional character than his or her own parent. In this way a character in a book or a movie serves as a vehicle for the child to displace his or her grief.

Abraham, age 8, had been very stoic in his behavior following the death of his mother from AIDS. For close to a year, Abraham spoke very little about missing his mother and refused to participate in any discussions about her that were initiated by his father or other close relatives. However, Abraham did become very involved in a television show in which the parent of a child in the show died. If Abraham was not able to watch this weekly show, he became very upset.

Miller (1971) explains that one way children deny death is by having a persistent unconscious fantasy of an ongoing relationship or reunion with the dead parent, even when they clearly know the facts of the parent's death. These reunion fantasies function to stave off the child's emotional emptiness. Children want so much to keep their mother and father with them that they may keep them alive in their minds.

Fantasized parents, Miller (1971) explains, also act as a control over the child's external behavior and actions. That is, the child will at times actually consult the imaginary parent for advice or for instructions. These fantasized or imaginary parents, if used adaptively, can serve almost as a transitional object, affording the child a less traumatic separation.

Immediately following the death of her mother, Betty, age 7, changed the name of her favorite doll to her mother's name. Betty began to take this doll everywhere including school. She was unable to sleep unless the doll was with her in bed. Sometimes Betty was observed sitting alone in her room talking to this doll. She would talk about everyday activities, feelings about friends, and school events. Betty's need for this doll continued but slowly changed in intensity over a 2-year period.

Arthur and Kemme (1964) have noted that children may also experience a change in their self-concept following the death of a parent. After the death, they often shift from feeling confident and secure to feeling hopeless, emotionally empty, and worthless. These children may struggle with intense feelings of separation anxiety, a sense of being abandoned, and a general state of uncertainty about their world and what to expect. These changes in a child's self-concept can be particularly striking when the death of a parent is AIDS-related. Most children, even at young ages, are somewhat aware of the stigma attached to the disease. After the loss of a parent, the child's sense of isolation and feeling of being different are often exacerbated by an awareness of the negative feelings associated with the nature of the death. The child who undergoes these changes will inevitably feel somehow diminished by the experience.

Children often experience a sense of guilt or feelings of culpability resulting from a belief that previous hostile or angry feelings they held about the parent caused the illness or death. Such feelings have numerous consequences for children's sense of self. Children, however, may be unaware of their guilt and other intense feelings and express themselves in indirect ways, for example, by becoming phobic. Nightmares and night terrors are frequent expressions of children's anxiety. Children may also become aggressive and impulse ridden, or, paradoxically, their behavior can become constricted and guarded (Arthur and Kemme 1964; Segal 1984).

Carmen, age 8, who had no history of sleep problems, began coming into her mother's bed each night following her father's death from AIDS. One night she awoke agitated from an apparent nightmare. She told her mother that she had had a dream that she accidentally killed a tall stranger who was wearing a jacket a lot like one that her father owned.

A myriad other, often subtle behavioral changes can also occur. Many of these are short-term or immediate reactions. Arthur and Kemme (1964) have noted these reactions generally refer to "essentially transient episodes signalling the ego's efforts to absorb the immediate shock" (p. 43). For example, upon learning of the death of a parent, children can sometimes appear withdrawn. This withdrawal may result from a need to internalize the anger about the loss. These immediate behavioral changes are often regressive in nature and vary depending on the child's age. Children may be very disorganized in their play, eat excessively, or stop eating. Younger children have been observed to start soiling, and older children may engage in frequent masturbation (Arthur and Kemme 1964).

These short-term reactions to the death, Arthur and Kemme (1964) note, can be followed by more long-term persistent changes in the children's personality if they unsuccessfully integrate the trauma of the loss. For children who may have suffered problems with "pre-traumatic personality development and organization," these risks for long-term consequences resulting from the loss exist. The child's capability to trust develops from the interaction and relationship the child has with his or her parents. This trust can be significantly disturbed by the death of a parent. In the long term, children can sometimes develop an inability to trust in relationships, leading to serious consequences for future adult intimacy and love (Arthur and Kemme 1964). If regressive behavior in response to the loss persists over an extended period, it will also impede children's development toward independence. As they move toward adolescence and adulthood, their ability to function increasingly autonomously can be significantly hampered. Or the child can experience a flight into independence too soon, fearing dependency on others for nurturance and growth.

The case example that follows illustrates some of the issues discussed previously concerning the latency age child's reactions to having a parent die of AIDS.

Michael, age 10, was informed of his mother's AIDS diagnosis about 1 year prior to her death. His father told him that his mother had contracted AIDS through her occasional intravenous drug use. Michael's reaction to his mother's diagnosis was initially hard to discern, as his outward behavior remained unchanged. However, he became extremely interested in the scientific aspects of his mother's disease and would ask his mother and grandmother medical questions. While his parents were open in their communication regarding the diagnosis and how his mother had contracted the disease, they emphasized to Michael the importance of not discussing his mother's illness with anyone outside the family. This need for secrecy both confused Michael and led to feelings of shame and humiliation.

A few months after learning of his mother's diagnosis, Michael began to have repeated somatic complaints, often developing headaches and stomachaches, which resulted in his frequently staying home from school. Remaining at home allowed Michael to be alone with his mother for extended periods. It soon became apparent that these physical concerns were related to a deeper worry Michael had about his own bodily safety. A secondary benefit of staying home from school was related to his recurring thoughts of his mother's illness and his worries about what his life would be like without her. Michael had a magical belief that if he were with his mother all the time, he would have the power to keep her alive.

After his mother's death, Michael was visibly sad. Behavioral changes both at home and at school soon became apparent. He changed from calm and compliant to angry and defiant. His school work began to suffer.

Michael began to see the school guidance counselor. After a period of time, he was able to tell the counselor about his profound feelings of loneliness. He described a feeling inside him that his mother was still alive. He explained that he often felt his mother's presence and that this feeling had a calming effect. He talked also about knowing that his mother was not alive, but also wanting to hold onto his inner feeling that she was still available to him.

Over time the counselor was able to help Michael see how his defiant behavior was related to how much he missed his mother, but also how angry he was at her for engaging in behavior that led to her death. The counselor was also able to help Michael understand that his wish to be reunited with her was normal. He encouraged Michael, with his father's and grandmother's help, to make a scrapbook containing pictures and other mementos of his relationship with his mother as a way of concretizing his ongoing emotional tie to her.

RECOMMENDATIONS FOR FACILITATING CHILDREN'S MOURNING AND ADJUSTMENT TO THE DEATH OF A PARENT

A variety of interventions help facilitate children's adjustment to the terminal illness or death of a parent. When the death can be anticipated, as with AIDS, it is essential to begin the process of preparing the child for the loss beforehand. Most of the recommendations offered in the following are relevant to the advanced and terminal phases of the illness as well as the post death phase.

1. *Provide the Child with Age-Appropriate Information.* Children's ability to understand illness and death depends on their stage of cognitive development. Consequently, they need age-appropriate information about the illness and death. For example, young children (say under age 6) typically cannot grasp complex concepts about causality. Nor can they understand the concept of the finality of death. It will have to be explained that "dead" means that a person's body has stopped working; it can't walk, talk or hear, eat or drink, or move any longer, and it will never be able to do any of these things again (Schaefer and Lyons 1986). Similarly, a report from the American Cancer Society (1986) on children's reactions to parental loss notes that because young children think in very concrete or literal terms one should avoid words or phrases that might be confusing to children like "taken from us," "sleeping," or "lost."

Somewhat older children are typically eager to know about their parent's illness and tend to use intellectualization as an adaptive defense. Thus they will request specific factual information about the disease, its cause and treatment. For example, a 10–year-old may ask, "What is AIDS and why does it make my mother so sick?" An appropriate answer for say a 9- or 10–year-old might be "Usually a person's body can fight off most germs. But when someone has AIDS, which is caused by a special kind of virus, her body gets very weak and she can't protect herself against these germs. So she gets all kinds of illnesses that make her very sick."

Children need an explanation of why the death has occurred, but generally these explanations should be kept short, simple, and honest (American Cancer Society 1986). They also need to have their questions about the illness, treatment, or death answered. With all children, but especially younger ones, explanations and responses may need to be reiterated. Children often repeat their questions as a way of being reassured that the answers have not changed or as a way of mastering their anxiety about the situation.

2. *Promote Open Communication About the Death.* Siegel, Mesagno, and Christ (1990) have pointed out that adults frequently feel it is best to avoid talking with children about a parent's serious illness or death. They mistakenly believe that in doing so they can shield children from the pain of the loss. In reality, it only serves to make the children feel isolated from family events. Further, the fantasies about events that children, especially young children, develop are often far more dire and upsetting to them than the real circumstances. Finally, talking to children about the illness and death creates the opportunity to discover misconceptions that can be rectified. The most common mistaken beliefs are that they are in some way culpable for the parent's illness and death, or that the illness is contagious or hereditary and that they or other family members will suffer the same fate.

Open communication about the illness and death should be promoted. Children should be encouraged to ask questions and express feelings—both positive and negative. Because a family member's HIV illness is often shrouded in secrecy, children may have concluded that this is something they should *not* talk about. And while there is a real necessity for selective disclosure in most cases, children need to talk to an informed person who can clearly and straightforwardly answer their questions. This may be a family member, a therapist, a school counselor, or the parent's physician. Children need to know with whom it is safe to talk about the illness and with whom it is not safe.

It may be necessary for the parent to initiate discussion about the illness with the child. Even young children feel the need to protect their parents and may avoid asking questions that they fear may upset them. As an example, a child may notice and worry that the ill parent is considerably weaker or more fatigued than in the past, but may not seek an explanation. A parent may have to acknowledge that what the child is observing is real and provide a brief, honest explanation.

Failure to provide the child with honest answers will only engender feelings of anger and distrust when the truth eventually becomes known. There is an understandable temptation to be evasive with a disease like AIDS, but this will not serve the child's best interests in the long run.

3. *Encourage the Child to Express His or Her Feelings.* Siegel, Mesagno, and Christ (1990) have noted that children typically need encouragement to express their painful and ambivalent feelings about the ill or deceased parent. They may need to be reassured that it is okay to feel bad or angry and that these feelings and thoughts are normal and do not have the power to harm their parents.

When a parent's illness is protracted and disruptive to family routines and the child's ordered world, the child typically experiences a range of negative feelings at various points. There may be anger that the illness has occurred ("Why did this have to happen to our family?"); anger toward the ill parent, especially if he or she is seen as having brought the illness upon himself or herself ("Why did he have to use drugs?"); resentment that life has been changed so much by the illness ("Why can't we still afford to stay in this apartment?"); resentment at the responsibilities the illness has imposed ("Why do I have to come home right after school to help care for Dad?"); and resentment of the stigma the illness threatens to impose on the family ("Why aren't my friends allowed to come play with me?").

Children will typically need permission and encouragement to report such negative feelings. They need to feel reassured that their feelings are common in their situation and that they are not bad for having them. Again, indicating that other children have reported similar reactions is reassuring and normalizes their experience.

Survival guilt may also be experienced by children, especially when a sibling or other family members have succumbed to the disease. Children may feel that they do not deserve to be well while others in their family have suffered so much. They need to be reassured that they do deserve to remain healthy and no amount of suffering by them would change the predicament or fate of others.

Children's communication styles are likely to vary by developmental age. Young children often have difficulty verbally articulating their emotions, fears, and fantasies. Having toys available—such as family puppets and doctor or nurse figures—may enable them to communicate through their play. As an example, a young child may express anger over a parent's death by repeatedly stacking up blocks and then destroying the structure by knocking them down. Drawing paper and crayons are also useful as children will often depict in their drawing their view of the ill parent, the family, or themselves. For example, a child may create a drawing of himself as small in proportion to everything else in the picture, reflecting his sense of helplessness and powerlessness in the face of the parent's illness.

4. *Address the Child's Security Needs.* Children often have very concrete and practical concerns about a parent's death. They will ask: "Who will take care of me?" "What will happen to me now?" "Who will make my meals and take me to school?" When plans have been made for the care of the child in the event that the mother becomes unable to care for him or her, the child should be offered reassurances that arrangements have been made to ensure that his or her physical needs will be met. Share the specifics when possible. When appropriate, include the child in the planning process.

Arthur and Kemme (1964) note the family disruption and sometimes dissolution caused by a parent's death, which causes children to view the world as unpredictable and may lead to pervasive fears of recurrent tragedy. Children may also hold common inaccurate beliefs that the disease is spread through casual contact. Thus they may worry that they or other family members are infected and will also die.

If the child is clearly uninfected, he or she should be reassured that he or she is young and healthy and will live a very long time. Young children need to be helped to understand the difference between a serious illness, which makes someone very, very sick, and the common everyday kind of illnesses, which most people get and are not serious or life-threatening.

If other family members are infected, a number of considerations need to be balanced in deciding what and when to tell the child. These include the child's age, his or her psychological resources and available social support, the nature and quality of the child's relationship with the infected individual, the infected individual's stage of disease and life expectancy, and how much other loss the child has already sustained. In all cases, however, realistic preparation needs to be balanced with the need not to burden him or her with the protracted awareness of anticipated loss nor deprive him or her of all sense of hope.

Once a child has been informed that a parent or other relative is infected, preparation for the possible eventuality of death should begin. That is, children should be informed of the parent's worsening condition at points of significant disease progression. While they should be informed that everything medically indicated is being done for the parent, they should also be told that the medicines and treatments may not work. However, they should not be deprived of all hope.

Because young children have a different sense of time than do adults, they should not be told that death is the expected outcome too early in the illness. If told, for example, that an uncle is going to die, a very young child is likely to interpret that to mean that the death is imminent and will likely occur in the next few days or weeks when in fact death may be many months or even years away. Even the older child who has a better developed sense of time should probably not be told too early to expect the relative's death because it would be extremely stressful to have to tolerate the anxiety and uncertainty that would be evoked by such an announcement over an extended period.

5. *Maintain as Much Stability and Consistency in the Child's Environment as Possible.* A family illness and death often necessitate changes in responsibilities, routines, living conditions, and even place of residence. Such extensive environmental change can deprive children of the feelings of security and comfort they derive from familiar routines and settings (Siegel et al. 1990). Relocation that requires a change of neighborhood or school can disrupt supportive friendship networks that could buffer the loss. Consequently, even if such disruptions are unavoidable, parents or caretakers should be counseled to try to maintain as much stability and consistency in the child's environment as possible. Even maintaining such simple routines as having meals at a certain time or going through an established bedtime ritual can reassure the child that all has not changed and that there is predictability in the world.

6. *Assure the Child that He or She Is Not Responsible for the Illness or Death.* As noted, on some level most bereaved children contend with the idea that their own aggressive behavior, misbehavior, or evil thoughts have been instrumental in the death. Children may also believe that if they had done something differently, such as helping the parent more at home, they could have prevented the unhappy outcome. Such magical thinking can not only contribute to a profound sense of guilt, but also create considerable anxiety that other negative thoughts or feeling can further harm the ill or well parent. Children may raise these concerns or openly express feelings of guilt. Whether they do or do not, they should be directly and unequivocally reassured that they were not in any way responsible and nothing they could have done would have changed the outcome.

7. *Help the Child Find Comfort in Pleasant Memories of the Deceased Parent.* Encouraging children to recall happier times with the deceased parent can remind them that even though the parent is no longer alive, they will always have their memories and the parent will always be a part of who they are and who they become. Silverman, Nickman, and Worden (1992) note that encouraging the bereaved child to make a scrapbook of pictures or keep some memento of his or her life with the deceased parent may assist him or her in emotionally separating from the lost parent while retaining a connection.

8. *Include the Child in the Funeral and the Rituals Surrounding the Death.* Adults often believe that the child should be protected from the rituals surrounding death and that attending a parent's funeral may be too traumatic for a child. While no child should be forced to attend a funeral or participate in rituals, the large majority can significantly benefit from doing so, if they are adequately prepared for what to expect. Weller et al. (1988) note that even atypical reactions to a parent's funeral have not been found to be associated with subsequent depression or other psychiatric symptoms.

Attendance at funerals helps affirm the finality of death. It also brings a closure to the events that have led up to it. Funerals and wakes also provide a socially sanctioned setting for the release of one's sadness and pain. Death rituals usually include comforting, assisting, and supporting the bereaved. Excluding the children from these rituals may deprive them of valuable family and community support.

Whether the child attends all or only some of the ceremonies associated with the death and burial, he or she should be prepared for what to expect to observe. What will transpire and why certain things will be done should be explained beforehand so that the child will not be startled, confused, or frightened by what he or she may witness.

9. *Respect the Child's Need to Maintain a Tie to the Deceased Parent.* Wessel (1973) explains that children often attempt to keep the deceased parent "alive" in their minds because of their intense need to possess a mother and

a father, especially in the first year of the loss. Silverman, Nickman, and Worden (1992) note that efforts to maintain a connection to the lost parent may include speaking to the deceased or keeping some object that belonged to him or her. Reunion fantasies may also be common and represent an attempt both to maintain a tie to the parent and to stave off an emotional emptiness created by the loss (Arthur and Kemme 1964).

Recent research by Silverman, Nickman and Worden (1992) on childhood bereavement has challenged the traditional clinical notion that the bereaved should be helped to detach emotionally from the deceased. Rather, it suggests that the focus should be on transforming these connections. Others (Sekaer 1987) have also suggested that a fantasized tie to the dead parent may be beneficial to the child, especially when no substitute parent is available for the child in reality. In such case a fantasized parent may be adaptive as a kind of transitional object until a new attachment to another adult can be formed.

CONCLUSION

That AIDS is still a virtually universally fatal disease dictates that loss and bereavement would be prominent psychosocial issues. That AIDS is a disease that often occurs among multiple family members suggests that resolution of the tasks of mourning by the bereaved may be considerably complicated. Further, the stigma associated with the disease and the resulting secrecy in which the illness is often shrouded may preclude open expression of one's grief, the accessing of psychologically "protective" social support, and participation in the societal rituals that can facilitate necessary grief work.

Clearly in the case of AIDS, there is a social dimension to the loss (reflected largely in the reactions from one's social group and the larger society) that tends to be absent in most cases of parental death from other causes. Indeed, it may be that it is along the dimension of social versus personal meaning of the loss that AIDS-related childhood bereavement differs most from other cases of childhood loss.

Most of the children who will be orphaned by AIDS will come from socioeconomically disadvantaged minority families. Parental death may be one in a series of significant stressors that they have had to confront. Others may be poverty, family or community violence, crowded living conditions, and physical abuse. Thus these children constitute a very vulnerable population. Every effort should be made to initiate intervention with them before the death. Identification of these children is often difficult because fears of the consequences of disclosing one's HIV-infected status lead parents to hide their diagnosis from their children or to instruct them not to reveal it to others. Clinicians working with HIV-infected mothers find that they are very concerned about their children's welfare and about the impact of their death on their lives. There is clearly a need for programs that ensure the family's confidentiality and yet make counseling services available to the children.

While we have focused on an individual counseling model, we believe that all of the principles for assisting children to cope with a parent's serious illness and death can be applied to a group setting. Clearly the usual benefits offered by groups, such as the provision of mutual support, the normalizing of experiences and feelings, and the sharing of information and coping strategies, could be realized by groups for children with HIV-infected parents or parents who have died of AIDS, assuming again that adequate safeguards of confidentiality can be maintained.

REFERENCES

American Cancer Society. 1986. *What Will I Tell the Children?* Washington, DC: American Cancer Society.

Arthur, B., and M.L. Kemme. 1964. "Bereavement in Childhood." *Journal of Child Psychology and Psychiatry* 5:37–49.

Baker, J., M.A. Sedney, and E. Gross. 1992. "Psychological Tasks for Bereaved Children." *American Journal of Orthopsychiatry* 62:105–116.

Bowlby, J. 1980. *Attachment and Loss* Vol. III. *Loss.* New York: Basic Books.

Camper, F., D. Langosch, K. Banks, G. Christ, F. Mesagno, R. Moynihan, K. Siegel, and L. Weinstein. 1991. "Children's Misconceptions and Distortions of Parental Illness and Death." Paper presented at the annual meeting of the National Association of Oncology Social Work, Monterey, CA.

Furman, E. 1964. "Death and the Young Child: Some Preliminary Considerations." In *Psychoanalytic Study of the Child* Vol. 19. New York: International University Press, pp. 321–333.

————. 1974. *A Child's Parent Dies: Studies in Childhood Bereavement.* New Haven, CT: Yale University Press.

Miller, J.B.M. 1971. "Children's Reactions to the Death of a Parent: A Review of the Psychoanalytic Literature." *Journal of the American Psychoanalytic Association* 19:697–719.

Osterweis, M., F. Solomon, and M. Green, eds. 1984. *Bereavement Reactions, Consequences and Care.* Washington DC: National Institute of Medicine, National Academy Press.

Schaefer, D., and C. Lyons. 1986. *How Do We Tell the Children?* New York: Newmarket Press.

Segal, R. M. 1984. "Helping Children Express Grief Through Symbolic Communication." *Social Casework: The Journal of Contemporary Social Work* 65:590–599.

Sekaer, C. 1987. "Toward a Definition of Childhood Mourning." *American Journal of Psychotherapy* 41:201–219.

Siegel, K., F. P. Mesagno, and G. Christ. 1990. "A Prevention Program for Bereaved Children." *American Journal of Orthopsychiatry* 60:168–175.

Silverman, P. R., S. Nickman, and J. W. Worden. 1992. "Detachment Revisited: The
      Child's Reconstruction of the Dead Parent." *American Journal of Orthopsy-
      chiatry* 62:494–503.
Weller, E. B., R. A. Weller, M. A. Fristad, S. E. Cain, and J. M. Bowes. 1988. "Should
      Children Attend Their Parent's Funeral." *Journal of the American Academy
      of Child and Adolescent Psychiatry* 27:559–562.
Wessel, M. A. 1973. "Death of an Adult: Its Impact Upon the Child." *Clinical
      Pediatrics* 12:28–33.

5

Adolescents and Parental Death from AIDS

Luis H. Zayas
Kathleen Romano

INTRODUCTION

From the time that injecting drug users and their sex partners began dying of human immunodeficiency virus (HIV)-related illnesses, adolescents have been made orphans by acquired immunodeficiency syndrome (AIDS). As the number of infected people continues to increase in minority communities, so will the number of adolescents orphaned by the disease. Perhaps no group of children in modern time has been more battered by the combination of social and familial decay and a devastating illness, coupled with the normal storms of adolescence. This group of youngsters may be the most damaged survivors of the AIDS pandemic.

For the most part, these are adolescents already burdened by a life spent with one or both parents heavily involved in drugs. They have experienced numerous disruptions, often going from crisis to crisis, along with their parents. In some cases, non-drug-using members of the extended family have provided respite for these children when necessary. More often, though, because the extended family is pervaded by drug use itself or because relatives do not want to be involved with their drug-using family members, the children remain with their parents, receiving occasional support from other members of the family in the form of food and clothing. Episodic foster care placement is a common fact of life for these youth.

In other instances, non-drug-using parents have been infected with HIV through sexual contact with infected partners or contact with contaminated blood via transfusions. If family life has been free of disruptions so common in drug-using families, the presence of an HIV-infected parent frequently initiates the spiral of family crises. A parent's or parents' certain decline in health and functioning, and eventual death, confronts the adolescent and his or her siblings.

Adolescents orphaned by HIV illness fall into three groups. The first consists of those uninfected youngsters whose parents died after the young person had reached adolescence. They are primarily children of injecting drug users and/or their sexual partners, but they may also be children of gay or bisexual men or of parents who have other risk factors for HIV infection. A second group is formed by those uninfected youngsters, orphaned as children, who have grown to adolescence since the death of their parent(s). Even if these youngsters had the developmental and familial resources to deal with their initial bereavement issues, an unlikely prospect for children in drug-using families, the changes of adolescence and the consequent search for identity tend to reactivate the feelings of loss and often require attention (Terr 1990). The third group is made up of those who are themselves HIV-infected, whether through maternal-fetal transmission or other means (e.g., transfusions, sexual abuse), and are now reaching adolescence.

In this chapter we focus on the first two groups, adolescents who are uninfected orphans and orphans-to-be of AIDS. We begin with a brief discussion of the developmental concerns particular to adolescence that may complicate those youngsters' reactions to their parents' HIV/AIDS diagnosis and subsequent death. Then we explore the issues surrounding HIV illness that make it different from other debilitating and life-threatening illnesses. Using examples from our own practices and those of our coworkers, we examine the psychological reactions of adolescents to parents' diagnosis of HIV seropositivity, AIDS, and death, and we provide illustrations of clinical interventions to help service providers develop a model of care for these youngsters. Some suggestions for clinicians' self-care close the chapter.

ADOLESCENT DEVELOPMENT

Because adolescent development is so broad and complex, not every aspect of it can or needs to be covered in a discussion of the impact of parental death due to AIDS. Our approach is to focus on adolescents' movement toward autonomy and intimacy (Erikson 1968; Blos 1962) as aspects of development that may be complicated by AIDS-related parental disability and death. This is particularly so because the move toward intimacy is entangled with adolescents' burgeoning sexuality, and both intimacy and autonomy are influenced by adolescents' moral development and need to make more complex moral judgments. The capacity of the family and cultural environment to serve as the test ground for this movement is particularly relevant to our discussion.

Adolescence transforms children's interaction with their parents in profound ways. Advancements in cognitive abilities allow adolescents to use higher levels of thought and reasoning in their interaction with their parents and to consider what occurs in the family despite being in its midst. That is, they are able to take an intellectual perspective apart from the family and think in terms of possibilities and alternatives (Piaget 1972). Posing a challenge to parental authority, adolescents begin to articulate their own conceptions of family roles, expectations, and responsibilities. They also define their own moral code, formulating moral judgments that may or may not be strictly in line with those of their parents, and that may be used to judge the parents themselves.

Recently, researchers have learned that this developing autonomy is not the same as total detachment from the family, especially not the freedom from attachment to parents and their influence (Hill and Holmbeck 1986; Steinberg and Silverberg 1986). Rather, the current perspective is that the adolescent move toward autonomy occurs within a family context, without necessarily bringing with it interactional upheaval in parent-adolescent relations. Not only does the youngster not detach from the parents and family, but he or she does not even desire to do so. What is desired, and usually achieved, is a renegotiation between the parent(s) and adolescent in which a sense of psychological autonomy can be realized. Gilligan (1987) points out that with the coming of age, the balance of power between adolescents and parents shifts and yields changes in the experience and meaning of these relations.

The feelings associated with the struggle for adolescent autonomy are those of sadness and loss. In effect, the young adult is killing the omnipotent, omniscient parent by internalizing many of the parental roles (Viorst 1986). No longer is the youngster totally dependent on the parents. Adolescents can exercise their own consciences in the decision-making process, they can look outside the family for emotional attachments, and they can meet many of their own needs. Like toddlers in the earliest separation phases, however, they are well served by the presence of adults who offer comfort, assurances, and advice, when asked, to fledgling adults without penalizing their attempts at independence.

With the onset of puberty, adolescents enter the childbearing generation, displacing the parents. This represents not only a dramatic shift in power, but an emphatic impetus for adolescents to solidify their own sexual identity. It may be the primary connection between the issues of autonomy and intimacy. The protection and security that come with intimate family life are shaken by this movement toward autonomy. Negotiating intimacy within the family means a change from the intimacy of childhood to the intimacy-autonomy balance of adolescence. Staying intimate with one's family while moving simultaneously away from it and toward intimacy with peers poses a dilemma for the adolescent: How can I be intimate with both when each side wants different, often conflicting allegiances from me? The problem for the adolescent becomes one of how to maintain supportive, consistent, continuous relationships with these persons that will, at the same time, allow some divergences.

As the adolescent becomes an adult person in his or her own right, the closeness lost in the family relationships must be replaced by the beginning stages of forming the nuclear families of the next generation. The "compulsory" heterosexuality of our society (Rich 1984) specifies just how those families are to be. Warm feelings that adolescents have toward their same sex peers become threatening in this intolerant environment, and adolescents need to gain some distance from these feelings in order to maintain an acceptable degree of psychological comfort. Moral prohibitions against homosexual behavior provide much of the feeling of distance and fit in well with the adolescents' need for a clear moral code of their own. The more uncomfortable they are with their affectionate feelings toward members of their own gender, the more rigidly and widely they need to apply this moral code. As a consequence, not only is homosexuality not acceptable for the individual adolescent, but the adolescent judges it as unacceptable for everyone. Exaggerated gender portrayals are a message to the world that this tough, cursing, spitting boy is a heterosexual man and that this seductive, heavily made up girl is a heterosexual woman. Adolescents who are unable to join their peers in denying the pull toward homosexuality in themselves suffer in isolation, furtively act out their sexual desires, or risk being ostracized and/or bashed by these peers for openly contradicting the gender stereotypes.

A crucial factor in the manner in which the developmental tasks of adolescence are negotiated is parenting style. With traditional parenting, in which parents want order and a sense of continuity rather than risk taking, adolescents tend to be more attached, conforming, and achievement-oriented (Baumrind 1987). In homes with authoritarian parenting in which parental power is restrictive and unquestioned, the process of achieving autonomy is more likely to be a battleground, generating problem behaviors among adolescents (Baumrind 1987). Families with democratic parenting are less guided by conventional standards, are more supportive of the adolescent's need for independence, and allow for some negotiation. The parents' capacity to adjust their perspective on the basis of the developmental needs of the adolescent and on the parents' own needs leads toward more adaptive functioning in the adolescent (Baumrind 1987; Smetana 1988).

When the family is able to permit conflict between members in the context of a supportive environment (Baumrind 1987; Powers et al. 1989), acceptance and understanding from parents (Hauser et al. 1984), and parental expressions of individuality and connectedness (Grotevant and Cooper 1986), positive outcomes for the adolescent's balance of intimacy and autonomy and involvement in the peer group are facilitated. Adolescents who have experienced individuated relationships within their families demonstrate more ability to maintain perspective in peer relationships and are therefore less influenced by the negative attitudes and behaviors of their peers (Cooper and Ayers-Lopez 1985; Cooper and Grotevant 1987).

Most developmental research and theory to date presuppose parental presence and do not take into account the effects of the physical and emotional unavailability of parents. Yet, in families in which drug use, and now AIDS, has spanned its history, adolescent development is qualitatively altered from what has come to be considered the norm. In both our clinical and personal experience with minority and/or economically disadvantaged families, we have often witnessed adolescents' being thrust into an earlier young adulthood than middle-class youth. Frequently, family dysfunction creates a need for the adolescent to confront social and psychological demands before their developmentally expected time. Older children are responsible for the care of their younger siblings, food preparation, and maintenance of the living quarters. In addition, bilingual children who have acted as translators for their non-English-speaking parents have been privy to information and part of family problem-solving processes far beyond their chronological age. As a consequence, even when the parent thinks that the adolescent may benefit from psychological help, he or she is less likely to put any pressure on the youngster to get it.

ISSUES PARTICULAR TO HIV/AIDS

Stigma

Many factors enter into stigmatizing HIV-related illness. In the United States, the immunological deterioration that came to be known as AIDS was first reported in male homosexuals, a group that was already highly stigmatized. The association between being gay and having AIDS was so strong that Ryan White, the HIV-infected teenager who fought so bravely to be allowed to attend school, was repeatedly asked whether he was gay. At the other extreme, when a colleague disclosed that she is a lesbian to her sister, the sister asked, "Aren't you afraid of getting AIDS?" Injecting drug users, another stigmatized population, represent the second largest group of HIV-infected people in the United States. Vilified as "junkies" and characterized as depraved, these drug users also became closely connected with the illness in the public mind so that many HIV-infected people, particularly minority persons from the inner city, were also suspected of having been drug users.

The second factor contributing to the stigmatization of people with HIV infection is the fact that the virus can be transmitted sexually. Though sexually transmitted diseases became less of an embarrassment after the openness of the 1960s and 1970s, most people still find it difficult to discuss sex openly in other than a joking way. To have a disease that can be transmitted sexually is thus an embarrassment, at the very least.

Finally, diseases that are thought to be nearly always terminal, such as cancer, while not exactly stigmatized, raise anxiety and cause others to withdraw from patients and their family members (Becker 1973). The ensuing silence engenders a feeling of shame in those affected, particularly in children and adolescents who do not realize that others are responding to their own fear of death. The isolation as others pull away leaves the individual and family feeling bereft of support.

Secrecy

To avoid discrimination, HIV-positive people hide their diagnosis from their families and communities. Older children, adolescents in particular, who know of their parent's HIV status, usually join the conspiracy of silence surrounding this disease. This tends to isolate the family, and the children within it, from possible sources of support in both the extended family and the community. Often, this secrecy leaves the adolescent without anyone outside the family, whose members are already involved in the emotional turmoil, with whom to share and discuss the illness and its anticipated aftermath of death, family disruption, feelings of abandonment, loss, and fear.

Paula, a 17–year-old, was initially required to keep her mother's HIV status a secret from her siblings and the rest of the family. Fortunately for her, however, her mother began to speak out courageously about AIDS discrimination in her community when Paula was 15 and her mother was a year into her drug recovery. Her mother's courage released Paula of her burden to keep quiet, and now she has a choice about whether or not to reveal her mother's HIV status. Now, according to her mother, they discuss the advisability of new disclosures, but the decision is entirely up to Paula. "I'm proud of my mother," Paula says, "and keeping the secret made me feel that I had something to be ashamed about. Not being ashamed makes us stronger as a family."

In cases where the secret is kept from adolescent children, parents often find that the youngster has known all along and has been keeping the secret to protect the parent. This is especially true when the parent has been battling HIV-related illnesses requiring lengthy hospitalizations and frequent clinic visits. Having to keep the secret deprives the adolescent of the opportunity to discuss the situation with the parent and to prepare for future bouts of illness and the prospect of the parent's death. Once the diagnosis is out in the open, however, the chances of helping the adolescent deal with it increase. Psychologists and social workers in HIV care need to provide individual, family and group therapies expressly for dealing with issues of disclosure. Often it is the clinician who understands why it would be helpful for the adolescent to know the parent's diagnosis and can help the parent appreciate the child's needs in an atmosphere of concern for the family.

Transmissibility

In the societal hysteria surrounding the AIDS pandemic, transmissibility has been confused with contagion. Children and teenagers are especially vulnerable to adopting such simplistic attitudes. Demb (1989) describes two youngsters who evidenced this fear of HIV infection. For one child, this fear, though initially unexpressed, was a conscious source of worry. For the other, it was indicated by her fear of both needles and condoms because of their association with HIV transmission.

Whether or not the adolescent mentions this fear, by bringing it up, the clinician can not only reassure the youngster, but also find out how much he or she knows about HIV transmission. Given the prevalence of sexual acting out in troubled youngsters, talking about HIV transmission offers another opportunity for these teenagers to be educated about how to protect themselves.

ADOLESCENT REACTIONS TO PARENTAL AIDS AND AIDS-RELATED DEATH

Bereavement

The most natural human reaction to death is, of course, bereavement. Children, like adults, go through the four stages of bereavement outlined by Bowlby (1980): denial, protest, despair, and resolution. Unlike most adults, however, children can stay in one phase of the mourning process for years (Terr 1990). In addition, they may be in both the protest and despair stages simultaneously, with the threat of despair fueling the degree of protest. Rodney, 13, is a good example of a youngster just beginning the protest phase after being stuck in denial for nearly 5 years.

When Rodney's mother died, he was 7 years old, and his sister was 5. They were both taken in by his mother's sister, Irene, and her husband, Jack—a young, caring couple with no children of their own. For several years, things went well for the new family. Rodney was a bright but quiet child who never mentioned his mother or the circumstances surrounding his entry into his new family. Irene's own natural reticence kept her from discussing her sister and the pain her sister's death caused her. Though Rodney's school grades never reflected his potential, he did well enough to keep his teachers and his new parents happy. When he turned 12, however, he entered the protest phase of mourning; things began to change and school became a battleground. Rodney's grades dropped dramatically, he refused to do his homework, and he even took to skipping school occasionally. As the pressure built, Rodney started arguing with his teacher and disrupting the class. By April, the month of his mother's birthday, Rodney had become so unmanageable in class that he was suspended from school.

In contrast, Eric, 16, was forced out of the denial stage by dramatic changes in his father's cognitive functioning. When Eric was 8 years old, his father, Bill, with whom he spent weekends, began showing signs of impaired immune functioning. By the time Eric was 10, Bill knew that he was HIV-infected, but he was well enough physically that he did not feel a need to disclose his status to Eric. A year later, however, Bill had a bout with toxoplasmosis. The seriousness of the situation became obvious on a weekend, when Eric was present, and Bill ended up being hospitalized for a little more than a month. After Bill returned from the hospital, Eric told his mother, Maria, that he did not need to maintain a room at his father's apartment anymore, and he would be staying with her on a full-time basis. When he visited his father, he wanted his mother to accompany him.

Bill and Maria agreed at this point that Eric should know the truth so that he could be prepared for the eventual loss of his father. In their discussions with Eric about his father's illness, Maria and Bill realized how frightened Eric had been by changes in his father's mental status. They were much more real to him than the possibility that his father would die. After a few months of seeing that his father was the same person he used to know, Eric began spending weekends with him again.

Gradually, Bill's cognitive functioning deteriorated. Eric denied that the changes were occurring, until, when Eric was 15, his father forgot his birthday, something he had never done before. Maria noticed that Eric seemed very depressed after this incident, but he refused to discuss it with her. He isolated himself from his friends and stopped paying attention to his schoolwork. Bill's partner, Irving, found an experienced adolescent therapist, and Eric agreed to see him.

With the help of the therapist, Eric began to mourn the loss of the father he once knew and to prepare for the physical loss of his father. In therapy, Bill's homosexuality, which had never seemed to be an issue before, became the focus of Eric's anger. The opportunity to express this fury to an understanding adult who withheld judgment on Bill's sexual identity broke the dam that contained Eric's sorrow. For 2 weeks, he cried every night, and he rarely visited his father. Recently he has begun spending time with Bill again, and with Irving and some of Bill's other friends. Eric stopped seeing the therapist but admits that "things might get rough again" when his father dies. If they do, his positive experience in therapy has provided the groundwork for him to be able to return to it again.

Depression

Depression, a turning-in of the psychic turbulence, is perhaps the most common reaction to the announcement of a parent's HIV infection, AIDS, and death. As occurs in most adolescent depression, the features of this dysphoria are variable. Withdrawal from family and social activities, sadness, isolation, moodiness, below- or above-average appetite, sleep disturbances, and inability to concentrate are all common. However, other manifestations of depression appear in the form of more externalized behavior, such as excessive risk-taking actions or provocativeness, that masks the depression. An associated manifestation of depression may be the initiation or acceleration of alcohol and drug use.

Acting Out

Acting-out disorders such as school behavior problems and disciplinary problems at home emerge. On one hand, the actual acting-out behavior by the adolescent may be corroborated by adults in the adolescent's environment, such as teachers, counselors, and adult family members. On the other hand, the family, particularly the HIV-infected parent or the responsible caregivers, such as aunts and grandmothers, may perceive that the adolescent is presenting unusual problems. These perceptions may be distorted by their own pain and suffering. At the extreme of acting-out behaviors may be anger that leads to violence and criminal activities. Swift and immediate intervention is certainly needed for the potentially self-destructive acting-out adolescent.

Overcompensation, or the "Superchild"

Some adolescents also assume the role of "superchild," in which he or she takes over caretaking roles for the parent and siblings, becomes involved in adult decision making, and extends him- or herself in household chores and similar activities, while attending school. Paula, mentioned earlier, is a good example of this compensatory reaction. As the oldest of five children, she works, goes to school, coparents her brothers and sisters, and provides most of the emotional support for her mother. The superchild can immerse himself or herself in these activities to keep busy and avoid facing painful feelings. A secondary motivation may be to get the attention and approval of the parent(s) that may have been lacking in the past. In addition, the behavior may also convey a sense of readiness to take on life's tasks in the absence of the parent.

Withdrawal

While the superchild becomes overengaged in a care-providing role in the family, other adolescents distance themselves from the fact of the presence of HIV in a parent. Running away or simply staying out of the house for extended periods during the day is a coping response that may be evident and developmentally related. Distancing not only provides time and space away from the parent and the pain but also may bring the adolescent closer to uninfected persons, such as a friend's parents (a form of "adopting a new, uninfected family").

Case Illustration

The case of Buddy brings together some of the developmental, emotional, and behavioral reactions.

Buddy is a 14-year-old Puerto Rican eighth-grader who lives at home with his mother and maternal uncle, both HIV-infected. His 10–year-old brother (Ralphie) and a 4-year-old sister (Linda) are also in the home. The three children have different fathers, and the extended family is scattered between the Bronx and Puerto Rico. Buddy's father lives in the Bronx but is not involved with Buddy.

Buddy's mother's HIV diagnosis worsened a preexisting chronic depression that she had apparently medicated with alcohol. She took a passive stance toward the illness and planning for her family. Although the announcement of her HIV status was made easily to Buddy and his siblings, it seemed that little further discussion occurred about their feelings and the impact on them. Buddy's mother did not engage fully with the social worker and psychologist available to her and her children at her primary care clinic, and she did not follow her medical treatment as recommended. Buddy and his brother were seen by the psychologist for several sessions, but family sessions with the mother were more difficult to arrange. At home, the two boys were expected to do many chores. They were basically unsupervised by their mother, but she berated them for their preference to be outdoors with friends rather than indoors with her. The boys complained that their mother was not interested in helping herself, unlike their uncle, who had taken a more stoic attitude toward his HIV status and focused on going about "life as usual" (including continuing to use illicit drugs).

Some notable developmental and behavioral responses by Buddy to his mother's illness were seen in sessions. Not knowing what to do with his diffused anger, Buddy tended to displace it onto his younger brother, Ralphie, often in the form of belittlement. As Ralphie acted out his desire for the protection and care of an idealized, helpful, and wiser older brother, Buddy could not tolerate the demands he felt coming from him. In the vortex of his own struggle with his mother's illness, Buddy's availability to his brother was limited, as was his mother's accessibility to him. Buddy himself sought help with his own hurt and fear yet could not move easily toward intimacy with others, such as a therapist, who could be there for him. In sessions, Buddy opened up his emotions enough to offer a glimpse of his pain and confusion but not enough to pursue them in any detail. He needed to be "able to do it himself" (autonomy) and was still frightened of intimacy with the male therapist, though he seemed to desire it.

The anger at his mother, which he tried to disguise, stemmed partially from his sense that she did not take care of herself enough to prevent the illness and then did not take care of herself as his uncle did. Instead, she jeopardized her life and, consequently, theirs by not following her medical regimen. Tied to this anger was Buddy's perception of the stigma that accompanies his mother's illness. Previously, Buddy had voiced concern that his mother's hanging out with the wrong people on the block would give her a reputation for being sexually promiscuous. After the disclosure of his mother's HIV status, Buddy was preoccupied with the stigma associated with it. Although Buddy denied that it was a concern for him, in sessions he mentioned that he knew that people in the neighborhood knew his mother was sick, but he would not affirm what was said on the street.

To counterbalance Buddy's negative feelings toward his mother, the therapist emphasized the positive affects of satisfaction and gratitude he felt toward his mother in providing for his essential needs. Attention was also given to several gifts from his mother—a crucifix on a gold chain, a ring with his name written handsomely, and frequent additions to his wardrobe—that she managed to buy him despite financial hardships and that were palpable demonstrations of her love. These issues become windows for discussing his feelings toward his mother, however fleeting the moments were in the sessions, and, to some degree, about his feelings for Ralphie.

Buddy also showed signs of envy that his sister had a father who agreed to take her when their mother died. Fueled by anger at his own father (an ex-convict who has neglected Buddy for his new family), Buddy skirted around the issue of envy by saying wishfully, "I'll be 20 years old when my mother dies and I'll be able to take care of myself."

Despite his mother's protestations that he was spending too much time outside the home, Buddy was engaged with some chums with whom he discussed God's existence and goodness, and the existence of the devil. Buddy's intimacy with these boys helped him deal, though indirectly, with his fear of his mother's death, his sense of impending loss, and his loneliness. The chums validated Buddy's self-worth in ways his family could not, but the stigma of his mother's illness prevented him from being able to share fully with his friends. In therapy, Buddy was given the opportunity, both individually and in sessions with other family members, to address the impact of HIV/AIDS on his life and his future. The therapeutic task was also to provide Buddy with a model of "surrogate parenting" that offers support, room for negotiation, and attention to his needs to help him navigate the adolescent passage of integrating his autonomy, intimacy, and identity.

INTERVENTIONS

Future Planning

To help with appropriate future planning, the clinician needs to ask many questions. First of all, are there any family members who are willing to take care of these youngsters? Despite very strong family bonds in both African-American and Latino families, these bonds can be worn away by years of drug use. Deception, manipulation, and outright theft may have been part of the pattern of abuse inflicted on the extended family by the drug user. In addition, the drug user's children may have been pawns in these encounters. Because of the children, family members may have given the drug user money for food only to find that it had gone to buy drugs. Children may have been dropped off with a relative "for a few hours" and been left there for days, weeks, and months. After these betrayals, family members are reluctant to remain involved. Even then, family members may be willing to take in younger children but may hesitate when it comes to an adolescent who is already angry and street-wise by the time placement becomes necessary.

A common feature in both African-American and Latino cultures, which can assist future planning, is the presence of an informal system of adoption. Among Puerto Ricans, the hardest hit of all Hispanics by the AIDS epidemic, this informal adoption system is known as *hijos de crianza* and involves the system of *compadres* (or coparents) (Mizio 1974). Among African-American families, Hill (1977) has documented the informal adoption system as a historical phenomenon that emerged to assure the survival of children and families during the time of slavery. For both Latino and African-American families, these informal systems of adoption are remarkable strengths that can be used in the process of the clinical work. Clinicians can expect to find extended family members, and even close family friends who might be considered "nonblood kin," willing to take in the adolescent and siblings. These networks of support are typically the first resource for the orphans.

Second, do the youngsters want to go with any of the family members whom they know? Future planning for the placement of adolescents requires their cooperation if it is to go smoothly. They have had their own experiences with the extended family. Some they like and trust, while others have treated them badly because of their anger at the drug-using parent. In moments of anger, for example, it is not unusual for a relative who is the actual or prospective caretaker to say that the youngster is "just like" the troublesome parent (Demb 1989). The transition to a new family is difficult for anyone under these circumstances, but it is nearly impossible for the adolescent who does not feel loved and wanted in the new setting.

Finally, are there any family members who are capable of providing a good home for the orphaned adolescent in particular? Pervasive drug use and family dysfunction are often not limited to the adolescent's own nuclear family. A relatively functional family that has raised a child from birth will often encounter difficulty when the child reaches adolescence. Placing a troubled teenager in a dysfunctional situation adds an enormous burden to the already struggling family. Drug use complicates the picture even more.

Clarabelle, 14 and debilitated by AIDS, was placed with her maternal grandmother after the death of her parents. There was no question that the grandmother loved and wanted to take care of this child, and Clarabelle wanted to live with her grandmother. Unfortunately, the grandmother was also allowing three of her adult children, all actively using crack cocaine, to live in her apartment. These adults consumed most of the food in the apartment, including the nutritional supplements that Clarabelle required to combat the wasting of her illness. When the visiting nurse assigned to the case realized what was happening, she reported the situation to child protective services, and Clarabelle was hospitalized so that her nutritional needs could be met. Even after it was no longer medically necessary, she remained hospitalized with very little chance of being placed in a foster home.

While many sources can be "mined" as resources for the adolescent, the extended family's initial enthusiasm to take in the adolescent and some siblings requires work. That is, sympathetic and enthusiastic family members may agree to accept the children without consideration of what short- and long-term effects this will have on their families. Likewise, taking in a more malleable younger child is very different from taking in a brooding, grieving adolescent struggling with issues of autonomy, independence, and parental loss.

Limitations to Planning

When neither kinship nor the culture-specific arrangements mentioned previously are available or feasible, what are the other options available for placing an adolescent? The answer is, unfortunately, not many. It is difficult to find unrelated foster families willing to take in an adolescent, whether an adolescent girl with her potential for pregnancy or an adolescent boy with his potential for physical violence, to name just two risks. According to Demb (1989), female adolescent survivors are at increased risk of pregnancy during the time immediately following their mother's AIDS diagnosis. A man-sized adolescent boy, who may have already gotten into trouble through his acting-out behavior, also stands little chance of being placed in an unrelated family unit. If the adolescent is part of a sibling group that includes younger children, it is not likely that a foster family can be found for the intact group. In such cases, the older youngster faces the loss of siblings in addition to the loss of a parent. Group homes then become the primary placement options for adolescents.

COUNSELING/PSYCHOTHERAPY

Difficulties in Engaging Adolescents

Most clinicians are aware of the difficulties in engaging teenagers in any counseling relationship, whether individual, family, or group therapy. It is not uncommon that the adolescent will resist or refuse engagement (Katch 1988) even when it is evident that those around the adolescent support the treatment intervention. The behaviors that can characterize the refusal may range from passive, compliant silence to active, physical refusal to attend the therapy (Zayas and Katch 1989). Indeed, working with adolescents has been considered a "fragile alliance" at best (Meeks 1971). Viewed developmentally, the difficulties of engagement emanate from the adolescent's tenuous identity achievement (Erikson 1968), the struggles with separation and individuation in which intimacy with an adult is frightening, fear of engulfment or submission to the adult when the adolescent seeks autonomy (Blos 1962), and the view of adults as substitutes to parental authority and control (Zayas and Katch 1989). Add to these the stigma of AIDS and the anticipated or actual loss of a parent and the problems of establishing trust are compounded.

Alternatives to Engagement of Adolescents

Often, the adolescents are not able to realize that the anger they are directing at the caretakers in their environment may be directly connected to their sorrow and confusion over the illness and/or death of their parent. In fact, they may not be aware of their sadness at all. Anger and "boredom" tend to be the predominant emotions expressed by acting-out teens.

When the teenager is not available for treatment (because she or he refuses to attend, or maintains a stony silence while there), the clinician must focus on the person or persons who present themselves for treatment. When Rodney was expelled from parochial school, his aunt, Irene, found both an individual and a group therapist who specialized in HIV-related issues for him. This was to no avail, however, as Rodney refused to attend.

The tension in the house was so great that Irene and Jack agreed to work with the therapist to tighten up their parenting skills.

Early on in the work, it became clear that natural reticence was not the only reason that Irene didn't talk about her sister. Irene's lingering resentment over her sister's life-style, coupled with her anger over having to disrupt her own life to pick up the pieces of her sister's, quickly came out. Because Irene thought that these were unacceptable feelings, she had not allowed herself to experience them consciously or to admit them to anyone else. Jack, too, had his own resentments. He had managed to remain unentangled with his own family by maintaining a distant but cordial relationship. Why, he wondered, had Irene gotten them both so involved? With the help of the therapist, they were able to discuss feelings they had labeled as "selfish" in an open and nonjudgmental atmosphere.

It also became clear that Jack had felt uncomfortable "butting in" on Irene's family business. This kept him from exerting a stronger influence on Rodney's development and from being involved in disciplining him. Work with the couple on strengthening their roles as heads of the household gave Jack permission to be an equal parent with Irene and relieved her of some of the burden she had been carrying alone. At the suggestion of the therapist, this now stronger parental unit began running weekly "family meetings" to discuss issues that had an impact on the smooth functioning of the family and to plan activities to bring family members closer together.

After four such meetings, both Irene and Jack reported that much of the tension at home had been relieved. There was less arguing over chores or curfews and more input from both Rodney and his sister, Kiesha, about how they thought things ought to be in the family. In the therapist's view, the family was no longer such a tentative entity. It was clear who the parents were, and it was clear that they were committed to each other and to the children. At this point, Irene and Jack felt that they no longer needed their parenting sessions, but reserved the option to return if necessary.

Final Words on Therapists' Stress

This chapter has dealt with the impact of AIDS-related deaths on adolescent survivors and the role of the clinician in helping the adolescent and his or her family resume its developmental course. A few words about the impact on the therapist of working with this group of orphans is in order. Until recently, there was little that could be done to prepare and help professionals working with HIV-positive patients and their families. The authors' experiences are not unlike those of other colleagues in this field.

For example, working with people with end-stage HIV disease for 3 ½ years in a municipal chronic care facility did not prepare one of the authors for the stress of dealing with the young families described in this chapter. After one particularly demanding day, she collapsed into a chair in her supervisor's office asking, "Can I do this work?" Wisely, he reframed the question as "How can I do this work?" For the other author, the early months of working with HIV and AIDS patients meant dealing with the arousal of irrational fears of infection, with the emotional and visceral reactions to the first sight of an acute case of Kaposi's sarcoma, and with the lightheadedness and nausea that occurred when he accompanied a physician friend on her rounds of AIDS patients on a medical service. The following are some suggestions for doing the work.

Since all families are dysfunctional to one extent or another (just as all families are functional to one extent or another), it is very likely that this work will stir up unresolved issues from the clinician's own past. Personal individual psychotherapy is an opportune vehicle for working toward resolution, as is individual supervision in an atmosphere that allows for the nonjudgmental exploration of countertransferential issues. In addition, Hummer (1988) points out that adolescents and children evoke a "universal countertransference" by virtue of their vulnerability and helplessness. A good supervisor will help the practitioner squelch the impulse to rescue in favor of helping the adolescent client develop the coping skills and judgment to deal with his or her situation.

In an atmosphere of unremitting sorrow, the ability to cry is often short-circuited. Sad movies and songs are useful triggers for releasing the build-up of tears, especially in the presence of supportive others. Organizers of "The Names Project" (commonly called the AIDS "quilt") seem to realize this. They provide squadrons of human comforters and boxes of tissues whenever the quilt is displayed. Viewing the quilt, like viewing the Vietnam Veterans Memorial, while essentially overwhelming, can break through the defenses against feeling the pain of our individual losses and allow the tears to flow in the context of a grieving community.

If the work environment is not conducive to allowing time for self-care, the clinician needs to lobby for this right. Periodic retreats devoted to "healing the healer" are conducted throughout the country. Major metropolitan areas have ongoing support groups for people engaged in HIV-related work. Consultants are available to run such groups in the workplace if there is a sufficient number of people involved to justify this. It should be cautioned, however, that in-house groups have their own problems. Developing a sufficient level of trust for the group to be helpful is much more difficult for people who work with each other on a daily basis and carry a lot of non-HIV-related baggage to the endeavor.

Finally, Winiarski (1991) talks about the need for clinicians to prevent the world of HIV from engulfing their lives. Leisure time should not be devoted to AIDS-related issues. Instead, free time should be spent on interests that provide nourishment and refreshment. Hiking, sharing dinner with friends, reading mystery novels, and viewing escapist movies are only some suggestions. The point is, there is much more to life than HIV, but this idea can get lost when one is immersed in caring for people with AIDS on a daily basis. Take time to look in another direction.

NOTE

Work by Dr. Zayas on this chapter was supported, in part, by National Institute of Mental Health grant MH30569 to the Hispanic Research Center, Fordham University, Orlando Rodriguez, Director. Work by Dr. Romano on this chapter was supported, in part, by Health Resources and Services Administration Special Projects of National Significance grant BHR 970025–01–0, Mark Winiarski, Principal Investigator.

REFERENCES

Baumrind, D. 1987. "Developmental Perspectives on Adolescent Risk-taking in Contemporary America." In *Adolescent Social Behavior and Health,* ed. C.E. Irwin, 93–125. San Francisco: Jossey-Bass.

Becker, E. 1973. *The Denial of Death.* New York: Free Press.

Blos, P. 1962. *On Adolescence: A Psychoanalytic Perspective.* New York: Free Press.

Bowlby, J. 1980. *Attachment and Loss.* Vol. III. New York: Basic Books.

Cooper, C. R., and Ayers-Lopez. 1985. "Family and Peer Systems in Early Adolescence: New Models of the Role of Relationships in Development." *Journal of Early Adolescence* 5:9–21.

Cooper, C. R., and H.D. Grotevant. 1987. "Gender Issues at the Interface of Family Experience and Adolescents' Friendship and Dating Identity." *Journal of Youth and Adolescence* 16:247–264.

Demb, J. 1989. "Clinical Vignette: Adolescent 'Survivors' of Parents with AIDS." *Family Systems Medicine* 7:339–343.

Gilligan, C. 1987. "Adolescent Development Reconsidered." In *Adolescent Social Behavior and Health,* ed. C. Irwin, 63–92. San Francisco: Jossey-Bass.

Erikson, E. H. 1968. *Identity, Youth, and Crisis.* New York: Free Press.

Grotevant, H. D., and C. R. Cooper. 1986. "Individuation in Family Relationships." *Human Development* 29:82–100.

Hauser, S. T., S. Powers, G. Noam, A. Jacobson, B. Weiss, and D. Follansbee. 1984. "Familial Contexts of Adolescent Ego Development." *Child Development* 55:195–213.

Hill, J. P., and G. N. Holmbeck. 1986. "Attachment and Autonomy During Adolescence." In *Annals of Child Development.* Vol. 3, ed. G. W. Whitehurst, 145–189. Greenwood, CT: JAI Press.

Hill, R. B. 1977. *Informal Adoption Among Black Families.* Washington, DC: Research Department, National Urban League.

Hummer, K. M. 1988. "Termination and Endings." In *Childhood Bereavement and its Aftermath,* ed. S. Altschul, 187–236. Madison, CT: International Universities Press.

Katch, M. 1988. "Acting-Out Adolescents: The Engagement Process." *Child and Adolescent Social Work Journal* 5:30–40.

Meeks, J. 1971. *The Fragile Alliance.* Baltimore: Williams & Wilkins.

Mizio, E. 1974. "Impact of External Systems on the Puerto Rican Family." *Social Casework* 55:76–83.

Piaget, J. 1972. "Intellectual Evolution from Adolescence to Adulthood." *Human Development* 15:1–12.

Powers, S. I., S. T. Hauser, and L. A. Kilner. 1989. "Adolescent Mental Health." *American Psychologist* 44:200–208.

Rich, A. 1984. "Compulsory Heterosexuality and Lesbian Existence." In *Women-Identified Women*, eds. T. Darty and S. Potter, 119–149. Palo Alto, CA: Mayfield.

Smetana, J. G. 1988. "Adolescents' and Parents' Conceptions of Parental Authority." *Child Development* 59:321–335.

Steinberg, L., and S. Silverberg. 1986. "The Vicissitudes of Autonomy in Adolescence." *Child Development* 57:841–851.

Terr, L. 1990. *Too Scared to Cry: Psychic Trauma in Childhood*. New York: Basic Books.

Viorst, J. 1986. *Necessary Losses*. New York: Fawcett.

Winiarski, M. G. 1991. *AIDS-Related Psychotherapy*. New York: Pergamon Press.

Zayas, L. H., and M. Katch. 1989. "Contracting with Adolescents: An Ego-Psychological Approach." *Social Casework* 70:3–9.

6

Latino Communities: Coping with Death

Esther Chachkes
Regina Jennings

INTRODUCTION

This chapter will discuss the experience of Hispanic/Latino children and adolescents who have lost parents, siblings, or other significant family members to AIDS. It is a survey of some of the cultural factors that specifically relate to bereavement, and it also touches on some general features that affect family functioning.

Latinos comprise approximately 8.2 percent of the population of the United States and are the fastest growing minority in the country, constituting the second largest minority at present. In 1988 the Latino population numbered 19.4 million and the projected figure for the year 2000 is 31 million (Ginzberg 1991; Council on Scientific Affairs 1991; Latino Commission on AIDS 1992). As the population has grown, it has also changed in name. As Gonzalez (1991) puts it, it was "Hispanics in the past two decades," but will be "Latinos in the next two." This difference is noteworthy. The term "Hispanic" or "Spanish-speaking" is not a racial or ethnic term. "Hispanic" people who come from Central and South America or the Caribbean may be white, black, Indian, or racially mixed. Some people from these areas may not even speak Spanish (Brazilians, for example, speak Portuguese). As a result of the imprecision resulting from the use of the term "Hispanic," the term "Latino" and its various gender-specific forms (e.g., "Latina" for a woman) have come into prominence. This is not entirely a satisfactory change, since in Europe all people whose language derives from Latin (e.g., French, Spaniards, and Italians) are called "Latin." Moreover, some Americans still prefer "Hispanic" (de la Vega 1990). In this chapter we will in general use the term "Latino," but will use "Hispanic" where the original source does so. Wherever possible, we will use more specific designations such as "Puerto Rican," "Mexican," or "Dominican."

Latinos come from a number of different countries, including Puerto Rico, Cuba, the Dominican Republic, San Salvador, Colombia, Ecuador, Peru, Mexico, and other Central and South American countries. The statistical breakdown by country of origin does not completely capture an accurate picture of Latino representation in the United States, nor does it fully capture the numbers of undocumented immigrants. Generally, Mexican Americans account for the highest proportion of Latinos in this country, Puerto Ricans come second, Central and South Americans are third, and Cubans represent a smaller number (Garcia 1991). A majority of Latinos reside in nine states, with over half living in California and Texas and 11 percent residing in New York State. In New York State, the largest number of Latinos come from Puerto Rico, but the number of non–Puerto Ricans is increasing at a significant rate. Latinos of Mexican background comprise the largest Latino group in the Southwest, particularly in California and Texas, while Cubans tend to be concentrated more in the Miami area and in New Jersey (Culturelinc 1991).

From 1989 to 1990, among all racial and ethnic groups in the United States, Hispanics had the largest proportionate increase (13.5 percent) in AIDS cases (CDC 1991). Mexican-born Hispanics residing in the South and West have the lowest rates, and Puerto Rican–born Hispanics in the Northeast have the highest rates (Diaz et al. 1993).

According to the CDC, Hispanics accounted for approximately 17 percent of the total U.S. AIDS cases (315,390) that had been reported as of June 30, 1993. By contrast, in 1988 Hispanics comprised only 8.2 percent of the total U.S. population (U.S. Department of Commerce 1989) Among cumulative U.S. male adult and adolescent AIDS cases, Hispanic men make up 16 percent, a proportion which is consistent with the Hispanic representation for all AIDS cases (CDC 1993).

However, Hispanic women and children are clearly overrepresented. Among cumulative U.S. female adult and adolescent AIDS cases, Hispanics make up 20 percent; among cumulative U.S. pediatric cases, Hispanics make up 24 percent (CDC 1993). In 1991, in the United States, the AIDS incidence (rate of new cases per 100,000 population) for Hispanic women was 7.5 times higher than the AIDS incidence for a comparable group of non-Hispanic white women (Diaz et al. 1993). In New York City, Latino women represent 33 percent of the cumulative adult female AIDS cases, and Latino children represent 37 percent of the cumulative pediatric cases (New York City Department of Health 1993, 7–11). These are dramatic figures and underscore the severity of the problem for Latinos.

The leading means of HIV transmission among Latinos continues to be associated with intravenous drug use. It is estimated that close to 50 percent of all Latino AIDS cases are due to intravenous drug use, either directly or indirectly. However, homosexual or bisexual behavior may be underreported because of the reluctance of Latino males to reveal this activity (Culturelinc 1991).

AIDS is the leading cause of death among Latinos between the ages of 25 and 44 in New York City (Chu 1993). The number of AIDS cases currently reported among adolescents nationally has been increasing. In 1990, HIV disease was the leading cause of death among Latino men aged 25 to 44 in eight states; it was the leading cause of death for Latino women in this age group in four states (Selik et al. 1993). Of the estimated number of children who are likely to be orphaned as a result of parental death due to AIDS, a disproportionate number will be Latino children (Michaels and Levine 1992, 3458).

CHILDREN AND BEREAVEMENT

The age of the child at the time of bereavement will influence the ability to comprehend death and loss and to express sadness. Critical to the child's management of the process are the availability of the family, the support network, both informal and professional, and the developmental needs of the child. Helping children cope with grief entails a knowledge of their perception of death and an understanding of personality, temperament, and their previous experience with death. Children are also significantly influenced by the reactions of those in their immediate surrounding and the responsiveness of other close adults (Wilfelt 1983). How others are handling the death may be critical to how a child will cope. Therefore, to understand the impact of death and the process of bereavement for Latino children we must understand the major cultural themes of Latino life.

ORPHANS OF AIDS AND THE SOCIAL ENVIRONMENT

The social environment in which Latino children, as orphans, experience their grief is of great significance. It has implications concerning the support, both formal and informal, that is available and how survivors will manage their emotional reactions to grief and the practicalities of their care. While many children come from caring and supportive social situations, a significant number of children orphaned by AIDS come from socially disorganized and poorly functioning families. In these families, social isolation, drug abuse, mental illness, poor housing, poverty, and discrimination have been ongoing aspects of their lives. This is particularly true for inner-city children.

For inner-city Latino children death is no stranger. In their neighborhoods people are shot and children are killed by stray bullets. Deaths due to drugs, crime, or street violence are not uncommon. Under these conditions, the risks associated with AIDS become just one more set of dangers that must be confronted; often the prospect of a future illness is less compelling than the survival needs of the immediate moment. Unlike children who experience the death of a parent within a supportive family background, they may never have had models of family life that offer support and nurturance available to them.

For many children family life has been severely disrupted. Parents may be trapped in violent and coercive relationships or have had episodes of involvement with the criminal justice system as a result of prostitution and other illegal activities. In addition, these children may have already experienced moving from one relative to another as well as several foster care placements. The loss of a parent may be only one aspect of a traumatic childhood that includes violence as well as separation.

MULTIPLE DEATHS

The psychosocial situation for orphans of the AIDS epidemic is made even more difficult by the unique aspect of this illness—the phenomenon of multiple deaths that often occurs within a family system or a peer group. Few other illnesses demand that the processes of grief, mourning, and bereavement take place in the midst of multiple deaths. It is not uncommon for families to experience the death of both parents and children. Mothers who are ill themselves watch with despair as their children die.

Prior to death, the family must struggle with many problems associated with the illness which are both medical and social. An HIV-infected mother may have had to care for an ill husband and sick children while meeting the needs of children who are not infected and dealing with her own illness. Under these conditions, it is very difficult for dying parents to plan adequately for surviving children or to help them manage their grief. The consequence of inadequate planning may be a continuation of separations and losses through foster care placements and sibling separations.

BEREAVEMENT

To understand bereavement, one must view it in its larger social context. Bereavement is culturally bound, subjective, and personal. People do not grieve alone; even in isolation they grieve as part of a community. Knowledge of how a particular community grieves helps professionals to understand how to be supportive to the survivor and what services will be of assistance.

There are obviously cross-cultural concerns in bereavement. All societies have customs related to death and mourning. Customs surround how people adjust to death, when they are permitted to remarry and to resume normal lives, and how losses are shared. All people have an emotional reaction to death, although the way it is manifested may differ according to cultural standards. Customs and beliefs dictate the view of the meaning of death, whether the dead are feared or revered, and notions about the afterlife. Customs also dictate how long one grieves and with what intensity (Rosenblatt 1975).

CULTURAL PATTERNS

In discussing the impact of culture on death and bereavement it is important to recognize that cultural patterns deal only with broad generalities. On the individual level there are many differences. An individual may fit a typical pattern or may deviate widely from expected cultural behaviors. Differences in education, life experiences, temperament, and socioeconomic class all influence the way in which an individual will adhere to cultural norms (Kalish and Reynolds 1976).

While most Latino groups have common cultural values and norms, there are differences between the various Latino groups based on country of origin and social history. There is an unfortunate tendency to ignore the cultural and political differences of Latinos; Latino groups are frequently lumped together with little regard to country of origin.

Latinos, however, have a strong sense of community. Country of origin and national identity are important aspects of self-identification and pride. National differences exist in diet, ways of life, political conditions, socioeconomic conditions, climate, and many other distinguishing factors (Novello et al. 1991).

The strength of the tie to one's country of origin is seen in the desire to be buried in one's homeland. It is considered a matter of honor for the family to provide for burial at home. It is not unusual for a family to hold a burial in the United States and then fly the body back to the country of origin when money is available to do this (Ghali 1977).

ACCULTURATION

The degree of acculturation is a significant factor in the social conditions of Latinos. Generations of Latinos born in the United States have different experiences and expectations from those who have more recently immigrated. The degree of integration into American society and culture, as in all immigrant groups, is a product of time and adaptation to mainstream values, expectations, and beliefs. Acculturation is also influenced by class differences, extent of education, and employability. Racial differences contribute as well; Latinos are of varying skin color. These differences are acknowledged with a range of attitudes and are frequently markers of social difference within the Latino community, even within the family.

Acculturation can cause conflicts. Immigration often involves not only a move to another country but also a move from a rural to an urban setting.

This can be very stressful, requiring a more demanding level of adaptation. In addition, since most extended families do not emigrate together, the normal support of the family group is often diminished. Furthermore, as family members emigrate at different times, the level of acculturation within the family can vary, with the potential of increased family conflict as members adapt to the mainstream culture at different rates. Integration into American culture, therefore, may not always be viewed as positive and in fact may be considered the cause of family problems (Curtis 1990).

Role strains for men may result from a lack of employment, particularly as a result of a move from a rural farming area to an urban area where different skills are required. Often it is easier for women to find work. This role reversal can produce a loss of male status and may lead to a defensive reaction escalating the need to display "macho" behaviors. Family tensions result when an employed woman is expected to defer to an unemployed male; she is expected to compensate for the shame he may be experiencing.

Acculturation as a process of transition frequently leads to cultural duality. Families must balance older cultural values while adapting to the newer ones imposed by experience with school, work, and the general society. There is often a feared loss of cultural identity. This dual perspective, then, can bring two cultural environments into conflict (Chau 1991; Garcia-Preto 1982).

Acculturation is also influenced by the ability to go back and forth to the country of origin. Puerto Ricans, for example, find it easier to "air bridge" back to the island because, as they are citizens of the United States, documentation and travel papers are not a barrier. However, almost all Latinos retain some connection to their country of origin. It is not uncommon for children to be sent back to be reared by grandparents and other relatives as needed while the parents remain in the United States. The "air bridge" phenomenon can also contribute to a sense of marginality as it becomes less imperative to integrate into American society quickly. This influences the continued use of Spanish as the primary language and may delay the assimilation process (Ghali 1977).

LANGUAGE

Not all Latinos speak Spanish, and their fluency with English varies. Some Latinos are bilingual but many second-generation Latinos do not speak Spanish well, and others speak no Spanish at all (Dillard 1983). Curtis found that many Latinos, however, favor bilingualism; English accommodates the needs of acculturation and Spanish maintains cultural identity (Curtis 1990).

CULTURAL VALUES

Despite these differences, there are key shared cultural patterns. Of significance in any discussion of the impact of AIDS, including death and bereavement, are cultural values associated with family life, communication, sex and gender roles, religion, and social integration.

THE LATINO FAMILY

The family in most cultures is the individual's primary social unit. Few social institutions are as significant as the family. *Familismo*, or "familism," is a prominent cultural value among Latinos. Familism refers to the "strong identification with and attachment of individuals to their nuclear and extended families; it involves strong feelings of loyalty, reciprocity, and solidarity among family members" (Soriano 1991).

Families handle illness in a variety of ways, and the psychosocial consequences of illness are influenced by the family's ability to cope with the illness and manage the different aspects of its course. Illness often has a profound impact on family life. Roles may change, and the nature and quality of relationships within the family may be seriously altered (Caroff and Mailick 1985).

A family's ability to cope is influenced by the degree of social and community support that is available. In most Latino communities, the family provides a network for protection and support for the individual. It is supported by an extended kinship system as well as the informal community network. Family ties include distant relatives, godparents, and close friends. Although there are some differences in Latino groups in the autonomy of the nuclear family, maintaining close relationships with the extended family is expected and highly valued.

In Mexican families, for example, closeness between parents and children is particularly strong, and less support is expected from the greater kinship system. In other Latino groups the extended family is a significant source of security and support (Kalish and Reynolds 1976).

However, all Latino families rely upon each other for emotional nurturance, and there is a strong sense of mutual commitment and obligation. The Latino family, therefore, considers the needs of the individual family member to be a family affair. It is not uncommon for individuals to consult other family members before important decisions are made, including those regarding health care. A particular family member may be informally assigned the primary decision-making role within the family. Frequently this role is held by a grandparent (Garcia-Preto 1982).

INFORMAL ADOPTION

Coparenting by the extended family system is accepted and viewed as legitimate. Children raised by a grandparent, parental sibling, or godparent are not stigmatized. Parents are not condemned when they utilize this surrogate arrangement for parenting. In fact, this is seen as a positive move because it prevents the children from being abandoned; room can always be made for an orphan or for a child of a divorce. Furthermore, this arrangement is viewed as an expression of the concern for children that is prized in the Latino culture.

This informal extended family system of adoption is frequently termed *hijo de crianza* ("reared child"). It is an understanding between natural parents and extended family regarding the rearing of children in the event the natural parents are unable to do so (Garcia-Preto 1982). Under this system, legal arrangements are not considered necessary and often there is no attempt to adopt legally (Moore and Panchon 1985). This informal system has at times been in conflict with the laws and regulations governing kinship foster care. Kinship foster parents often resent the supervision of foster care or governmental agencies and do not adhere to certain regulations which may not appear to be culturally acceptable, including limiting the visitation of natural parents because, for example, they are drug users (Sanchez 1992).

For most Latino orphans of the AIDS epidemic, the maternal grandmother or aunt becomes the mother surrogate and provides the protective web of family life. The Latino woman holds the family together, bonding family members through affection and caregiving. However, these grandmothers are often poor women, aging and overburdened. Caring for a grandchild may be an unwanted or difficult burden, an intrusion into family life. The children may be strangers within the family, isolated by the unacceptable behavior of their parents and the shame of drug addiction and AIDS. For many of these grandmothers, who are not part of the kinship foster care system or known to other agencies, few services and little information are available, especially in Spanish. If the orphans they are caring for are also HIV-infected, they may be unprepared to handle the basic aspects of caregiving around an infectious illness.

Godparents also carry responsibility for children, generally to offer help in times of trouble, sometimes economic or other types of personal assistance, even acting as a guardian when needed. However, godparents may be unprepared to take on the burden of total care for an orphan.

In addition, other relatives, generally aunts or uncles, who have avoided drug use and who have been able to maintain socially acceptable life-styles, may resent having to take care of surviving children of their less fortunate siblings.

The ambivalent feelings held by other key family members toward the rearing of these children, despite cultural expectations to do so, will have psychological consequences for the child. This ambivalence must be shouldered by the child, along with the problems usually associated with separation and loss that are difficult for children even under the most favorable circumstances. When the surrogate support system breaks down, the child is often abandoned, as the case of Marta illustrates.

Marta is 14 years old and was recently diagnosed with HIV infection. Her mother was an IV drug user, killed during a drug deal when Marta was 6. Her father died of AIDS 5 years later. Both parents were from Puerto Rico. Marta has four half-siblings but they live in Puerto Rico and she has no contact with them. Marta's mother had three siblings—two sisters and one brother. After her mother's death, she lived briefly with one of her aunts. As Marta began to show signs of her illness, both aunts, frightened of the disease, felt they could no longer care for her. She then was sent to live with her elderly *Madrina* (godmother). Without support from her other children, her *Madrina*, who was deeply religious, enlisted the help of church members. They provided, in addition to spiritual support, help with chores and the care of Marta. At the same time, Marta's uncle, also an IV drug user, returned to live with his mother. However, he continued to deal drugs from the home and stole money, medications, and even Marta's food supplements. Visiting Nurse Service reported the case to the Child Welfare Administration, who placed the family in a newly established shelter for AIDS families. While she was living there, her *Madrina* died suddenly of a stroke. Marta's aunts were unwilling to take her home, afraid for their children and the risk of contagion. Marta was sent to a pediatric long-term care facility. Marta is withdrawn and depressed. She shares little with the hospital staff. She has had a short and sorrowful life of poverty and loss and has been the object of fear, social rejection, and family shame. Her fondest memories are of her *Madrina*'s church companions and members of the Santeria community, who visited her, prayed over her, lit candles, and burned incense in the hope of her recovery. Now she awaits her own death with little respite from her despair.

GUILT AND SHAME AND HOMOPHOBIA

Intimate matters are often not discussed within the family and even less frequently with individuals outside the family system. Issues that cause guilt or shame, in particular, are not easily shared. Strong emotional reactions may be expressed without revealing the real source of distress. Although more religious family members may talk to the parish priest about shameful family issues, to seek support outside the family may be viewed as compromising the family's pride and dignity (Dillard 1983). Living up to the family's expectations and maintaining its unity are of great importance. Behavior that might cause family dishonor may be kept secret.

Homosexuality and bisexuality often are not acknowledged because doing so would bring dishonor to the family. There are strong cultural prohibitions against such behavior. In Latino culture, with its polarization of male-female roles and emphasis on *machismo* and *marianismo* ("Mary-like" behavior), homosexuality is not acceptable (Culturelinc 1991; National Commission on AIDS 1992). Many Latinos identified as openly gay have experienced discrimination and rejection by their families and in their communities. As a result, AIDS, linked to homosexual behavior, is highly stigmatized and handled with shame and with secrecy (Stuntzner-Gibson 1991). There is often no communication about the illness, and not much is shared within the family.

When there is little discussion in the family and when children, in particular, are excluded from conversations concerning the illness, children may not be prepared for the death of their parent and for the circumstances of their life after this death. The family's shame and guilt can also impede connections to the community. The secrecy of AIDS can hamper the normal involvement of the extended family, which is a prime source of comfort and support.

Marina's case illustrates issues of communication, shame and secrecy.

Marina is 10 years old. She lives with her grandmother but was raised by an uncle, Jesus, who died of AIDS when she was 9. She does not understand why he died and she misses him greatly. In response to this loss, she suffers from nightmares and wakes up asking for him. She believes he died of meningitis. Jesus was a cocaine and heroin addict and he was bisexual. Although he had been an addict for many years he maintained a fairly stable life. The family supplied him with money and kept his drug use secret. He was a good parent surrogate, loving and kind.

Marina is separated from her parents. Her father died many years ago as a result of a knife wound. The details of this event, shrouded in secrecy, have also not been discussed within the family and Marina knows very little about her father. Her attempts to get information are treated as inappropriate requests and too personal. Marina's mother is HIV-infected. Because she is a drug addict, the family believed that she was not able to care appropriately for her child. They decided that Marina should be brought up by her maternal grandmother. Although Marina's mother lives elsewhere, she is connected to her child, buys her clothes, and sees her frequently. Her drug addiction and HIV infection, however, are not discussed with Marina. Marina has experienced separation from all the significant parental figures in her life except her grandmother, and yet she knows very little about why these separations occurred. She has had little opportunity, therefore, to express her worries and concerns and lives with a confusing picture of family loss. She fears further losses and cannot talk about her anxiety as she is never given specific details and information.

GENDER ROLES

In marriage, men and women carry different roles, and gender role differences are pronounced. Leavitt and Lutz (1988) describe the differences in socialization patterns of male and female children, which emphasize modesty and protection for females while indulging males. Male rebelliousness is expected, and interaction with the larger community is encouraged for men but not for women.

The Latino family is patriarchal and the husband or father is the authority and prime decision maker (Garcia-Preto 1982). As such, he is expected to be dignified, hard-working, and "macho." Latino cultures typically are based on the concept of *machismo*, which emphasizes the dominant position of men in the social order. Women are generally expected to remain at home and keep the family together, while the man has much more freedom and is not expected to take on household or child rearing chores.

A double standard of sexual behavior also exists; men are allowed to have extramarital affairs, but women are not. According to cultural norms, sex is defined by masculine demands and expectations. *Machismo* demands virility and sexual prowess. Women are expected to remain monogamous and silent partners with little power in the matter of sexual relations. This is particularly significant in the context of AIDS, because it affects the women's ability to influence safer sexual practices. Men, in general, may reject using a condom, equating its use with prostitution. Women may feel unable or unentitled to demand that a condom be used. In addition, it is often the woman who is blamed for infecting the male if both are HIV positive, even in cases where the evidence suggests the reverse. The woman is expected to accept and support this explanation (Soriano 1991).

In marriage, as well as outside marriage, intimate matters are generally not discussed. Sex is a taboo topic, considered private and personal. Sex education is generally not provided for children in the home, and women are not expected to know much about sex. Furthermore, because bisexual or homosexual behavior is not acceptable, discussions about these behaviors are considered taboo as well (Marin 1990).

However, the concept of *machismo* does incorporate the man's responsibility to protect his family and to provide adequately for them. Protection also includes protection from seduction. Women are reared strictly and the concept of *Marianismo* expects the woman to be submissive and obedient. However, women are expected to be sexually attractive and to present themselves in such a manner. This often results in a seductive manner of dress and in great attention to personal appearance.

The "good" woman also treats motherhood as central in her life and devotes herself to her children. Motherhood is venerated in Latino culture, and children are very important to both women and men. The woman who sacrifices her life for her children fulfills the mothering role in a culturally appropriate manner (Ghali 1982).

INTERPERSONAL RELATIONSHIPS

In addition to mores associated with family and gender, several other important cultural attitudes are significant in interpersonal relationships and influence behavior. *Simpatía* is an attribute that relates to the importance of politeness, respect and diplomacy in personal relationships. Direct confrontation and criticism are considered inappropriate behaviors. Latinos will frequently appear to agree with someone despite a different opinion in order to offer a *simpático* response. The concept of *personalismo* is the preference for relationships with others who are known personally in a social group. Respect is central in all relationships and influences how people relate to others in regard to age, gender and social class. Showing personal respect is critical (Garcia-Preto 1982). *Respeto* extends to authority figures as well and can lead to a deferential approach to those persons (Marin 1990; Ghali 1982). All these values, which influence interpersonal relationships, are critical aspects of the relationship between professional helpers and the Latino client.

COMMUNITY

For most Latinos, community and neighborhood are important sources of social support. The community complements the family, and it is not uncommon for Latinos to cluster geographically. However, the presence of strong community ties presents a social pressure, which can reinforce the power of shame and guilt for unacceptable behavior—an important factor for persons with AIDS (Delgado and Humm-Delgado 1982).

RELIGION

Just as community complements the family, religiosity enriches communal life. Most Latinos are Catholic, although there is a significant number of Protestants, often from fundamentalist sects. The norms of Catholic behavior, including attitudes toward sexual behavior, sex education, birth control, and homosexuality, are powerful influences in Latino life. Religion also influences fatalistic attitudes. Latinos view illness as "God's will," brought about by previous or current sinful behavior or as a result of suffering that is intrinsic to the human condition. One of the common responses to illness is the attribution of the illness to divine punishment (Kalish and Reynolds 1976). Tina's case illustrates this.

Tina believes her mother has AIDS because of "God's punishment." The conflict surrounding her reaction to her mother's impending death, both her anger and her sorrow, is painfully obvious. She wants to forgive her and to save her mother. Yet she is angry that her mother's life-style has brought such pain to the family and that she and her siblings have been so unprotected. Tina is the eldest of four children. She is 19 and has three siblings: Estrella, Carlitos, and Sara. When she was little, Tina's uncle sexually abused her. She never told anyone. This uncle subsequently died of AIDS. Now her mother is dying of AIDS, and Tina believes that both her uncle and mother are being punished for what was done to her. Estrella, Tina's sister, believes she can also save her mother's life. She believes that if she does very well in school, God will reward her and allow her mother to live. She believes her hard work and accomplishment can save her. Estrella lives with her grandmother, who is ill and aging. Estrella and her grandmother talk about AIDS and their family. However, her grandmother supports the idea that her daughter's death is God's will and fatalistically accepts it.

HEALTH BELIEFS

Health beliefs are also culturally determined. Latinos tend to adhere to a view of health that they believe results from the interaction of emotional, physical, and interpersonal situations. An upset in one aspect can result in physical illness. The hot-cold theory of good health in which there is a "balance between the body humors" is a well-known Latino belief system. Food and medicines are labeled as "hot" or "cold," and a proper maintenance of temperature is important in healing (Delgado and Humm-Delgado 1982).

Many Latinos seek alternative supports to traditional medicine. The *santeria* (*espiritismo* or *curanderismo*) is a complex form of beliefs and practices that encompasses aspects of body, spirit, and mind. *Curanderismo* assists the individual in alleviating anxiety and provides protection and guidance. The *santero* may use herbs, candles, or dietary advice and provides an important cultural function. *Espiritismo*, or spiritualism, is an amalgam of Catholicism and native beliefs, originating over 500 years ago at the time of the Spanish conquest. The *santero* serves as a "folk doctor" and is often used in addition to traditional medicine. The *botanica*, where herbs and candles are sold, is a visible presence in the *barrios* throughout the country (Rivera 1990).

DEATH

The view of death is basically similar in all Latino groups. There is a fatalistic acceptance of death; it is sorrowful and tragic but unavoidable. Among Puerto Ricans, the death of an infant is particularly tragic because of the high value placed on children. According to Garcia-Preto (1991), Puerto Ricans used to dress the infant in white, paint its face to look like an angel, place flowers around the coffin, and sing songs to hail the baby's arrival in heaven. She notes that the death of young parents, leaving children who must be cared for, is also considered especially tragic.

Concepts of an afterlife include the idea of spiritualism—a world of spirits (good and evil) that surround the known world and that can influence the lives and the behaviors of individuals. After death the individual joins the spiritual world and may in fact have greater power and increased well-being (Garcia-Preto 1982).

The rituals surrounding death have little variation. Mourning and burial rituals are essentially Catholic in origin. Intense displays of emotion from Puerto Rican men and, especially, women at the time of death, during the viewing, and at the funeral are expected. These expressions of grief are expected to end after the burial, as the mourners accept the death (Garcia-Preto 1991). There are differences in rituals for Pentecostal sects, such as a closed rather than an open casket and a lesser degree of expressed grief. In some Protestant sects, a display of too much grief reflects a lack of faith in God.

Latinos rarely choose cremation and value burial where other family members are interred. After burial the family goes to the home of the deceased for prayer services. There are at least 7 days of prayers, during which the rosary is said. This provides a time of contemplation and family support. It also mobilizes the survivors, who must provide food for the mourners. Mass is said monthly for about a year and novenas (prayers to the saints) are also said. Close family members show respect for the dead by wearing black for a period of 1 year, by saying nothing negative about the deceased, and by making annual visits to the cemetery. Because of the high value placed on gathering for the death and funeral, and on resolving old conflicts, a family member who is not able to be present may have difficulty in resolving the loss (Garcia-Preto 1991).

LATINO CHILDREN AND DEATH

Although for children, the death of a parent is perhaps one of the most compelling and sorrowful events that they will experience, in the Latino family and of there is often very little discussion about death and the needs of children to mourn. Children often play a peripheral role in the preparations and activities of the mourning processes. Although they may be taken to the burial service, they are not expected to show the same level of emotion as adults. When a parent has died, children may be told that the parent is in heaven with God, watching over them and guiding their caretakers (Kalish and Reynolds 1976; DeSpelder and Strickland 1987). This may be a literal belief including the idea that the dead send messages. The cultural attitude toward death supports an underlying acceptance of death and a deep belief in an afterlife. As a result, while there is an acceptance of strong emotional reactions and the rituals of burial allow for a time of family comfort, there is little concern that children will experience psychological problems as a result of this loss.

Jessica is an example of a child with psychological reactions to death who is unable to talk openly about these within her family.

Jessica, age 9, is the oldest of two children living with her mother and father and a 2-year-old sister, Norma. Norma was diagnosed with HIV at approximately 10 months of age after a series of infections. Norma's parents, Jose and Maria, have been together for 4 years. He works as a grocery clerk, and she is a homemaker. Neither has a history of drug or alcohol abuse, and they have lived relatively stable lives. They are close to their respective families and have many friends both in the United States and in Puerto Rico, their country of origin. After Norma's HIV infection was discovered, both parents were tested and both were found to be HIV-infected. Jose suspects that his risk factor was a previous heterosexual contact, prior to his relationship with Maria, and that Maria was subsequently infected and then passed the virus on to Norma. Jessica is not infected and will be the only surviving member of her nuclear family. The specter of impending death permeates family life.

Jessica is a bright, articulate, creative 9-year-old who has always done well in school and has had successful social relationships. Her parents have not been able to talk to her about their HIV status or about Norma, although they are aware of her deep concern and worry. Maria reports that Jessica has become increasingly dependent and clings to her in a way that she never did previously. Jessica remains unable to express her fears, and Maria is worried about her. However, she becomes very depressed and upset when she thinks about the issues related to this illness in the family and cannot easily talk about them.

As with all children who know there is a family secret, and that it somehow is going to have a major impact on their lives, Jessica needs to be reassured about her own safety and her future. She is very aware that there has been a change in her family functioning, despite her parents' attempts to "keep things normal." The family has become involved in counseling and with the support of social workers and peers, their ability to talk openly about what is happening and to plan for the future is improving.

COPING

The surviving child has often had to face a number of overwhelming losses and a cycle of repeated rejections usually well before the actual death of the parent. Illness, drug use, poverty, and all the deprivations of inner-city life have made abandonment and neglect central themes in their young lives. The cycle of foster care, moving from one relative to another, and watching the deterioration of family life is a familiar experience for many of these children. In some families the experience of rejection is intensified by acts of violence, including domestic violence and child abuse.

Situations of drug use may have already disrupted normal cultural patterns in which families cared for each other. Coping skills that usually would be available to the family are lessened, increasing the likelihood of hopelessness, alienation, and social isolation. When the Latino desire to maintain the family as a self-sufficient unit within an unstable world is unattainable, the locus of emotional support is seriously compromised.

In the drama of death, the surviving child can feel abandoned and forgotten. Children defend themselves against these feelings in a variety of ways. Reactions to the trauma of death and of multiple losses run the gamut: acting out, running away, drug use, withdrawal, depression, poor school performance, truancy, and unmanageable behavior are often the strategies used by children to express their pain.

Some children, worried about foster care placements and eager to please rather than experience another loss, may manifest overly compliant behavior. In other cases, the trauma and the stigma are internalized. Children may feel that they are somehow bad, tainted by the unacceptable behavior of their parents and siblings. They are torn between concern and sorrow for their parents and blaming them for their illness.

The case of Filio is an illustration of this.

For Filio, a 16–year-old orphan, running away from kinship foster care seemed to be the only option open to him. Filio did not want to accept the reality of his parents' death. He believed that his parents had not died but were hiding from him "in one of the city parks." He had very little information about his parents' illness and death, and the response of his extended family was shaped by their shame. He did not have a good relationship with either of his drug-abusing parents. He suffered a great deal of physical abuse but this abuse was apparently not reported. He remained with his parents until their death, although he spent increasing amounts of time with a maternal cousin as his parents became more debilitated.

After their death he went to live permanently with his mother's cousin, who took him in as expected in Latino families. However, she resented the burden of his care and was unable to control his behavior. After he ran away, Filio survived as a homeless runaway for two years. During this period of time he became a cocaine user and supported himself through bisexual prostitution. He first came to the attention of the Child Welfare Administration when he impregnated a 14–year-old girl, Patricia. Patricia was very fond of him. Despite her youth, the experience of love and comfort enabled Filio to begin to make significant changes in his life.

Filio is one of the lucky ones. A supportive network of caring professionals became strongly engaged on his behalf. He is now in drug treatment and has been involved in counseling sessions, which have enabled him to confront members of his extended family. He desperately wanted to know about his family, particularly his father, in order to further the healing process. He was finally told that his father had been bisexual. The family was too ashamed to make that admission at first. His father's bisexuality and HIV infection were hidden by the family. Filio had only "bits and pieces" of information gleaned from overheard conversations in hushed tones. He never fully understood until it was too late what was wrong and had no ability to say a proper good-bye or to share his worry and fear. The cultural prohibition in discussing sex, the homophobic reactions of his extended family and the shame of his community deprived him of a needed bereavement and mourning experience.

Not all orphans of the HIV epidemic come from socially disorganized situations, and many have received the support and care they need to help them manage the chaotic world of death, disease and loss. There are children who come from close and loving families who, despite the consequences of the illness and low socioeconomic status, fight heroic battles to keep their family together and to manage throughout the course of the illness. The courage of many dying mothers is well documented by professionals who have helped them to make last-minute custody arrangements, while keeping their family together as long as possible. Two cases illustrate this situation:

Lydia died 2 years ago after a third episode of *Pneumocystis carinii* pneumonia (PCP). She left three children, who now live with her family in Puerto Rico. For the 2 years prior to her death Lydia struggled to cope with her illness and to maintain her family. Despite her illness and severely debilitated state, she kept an immaculately clean home. The children had been made aware of the fact that their mother was dying and was very ill. She died on Christmas Day. Lydia lived with her boyfriend, Antonio, who remained with her until her death. Her family did not approve of her relationship with Antonio because he was younger and also had AIDS. The children's father had died previously of AIDS. After Lydia's death Antonio became severely depressed and suicidal, and the children were at first placed in kinship foster care with an aunt and then sent to other family in Puerto Rico. These arrangements were made by Lydia before her death. Despite the family's initial estrangement, they have now rallied to provide care for the children and have even accepted Antonio.

Margarita and Reynaldo had three children, a 6-year-old boy and infant twins, one of whom died at the age of 9 months of pneumonia. As a result of this death, Margarita was tested for HIV infection and was found to be positive. She was apparently infected by a previous partner. The second twin was also infected and has recently died. Margarita is expected to die shortly, leaving Reynaldo and their 6-year-old son as the only survivors of this family.

Reynaldo is a carpenter and has been steadily employed. He is a loving husband and father, and both he and Margarita had hopes of building a strong family life, buying a small house, educating their children, and leading a middle-class life. They were pulling themselves out of the *barrio* and into a more financially secure situation when Margarita was told of her diagnosis. Reynaldo is emotionally devastated. He is having difficulty dealing with so much loss. He has a supportive family and has looked to them for help. His 6-year-old son has become withdrawn and obviously frightened. Reynaldo is aware of his son's pain and has requested professional help for him at the same clinic where his wife is receiving mental health treatment. He has also looked to his family to provide support and care for his child. Currently he is overwhelmed and in crisis.

CLINICAL CONSIDERATIONS

Because AIDS is still relatively new, findings in the literature are limited, particularly those addressing the needs of Latino orphaned children. Clinical settings that cater to Latino clients often must construct their own service provisions with newly defined treatment goals in mind.

Comfort with counseling interventions is highly dependent on the level of acculturation and the support of the extended family. Less acculturated Latino clients may never have sought help from outside sources previously and may find it difficult to disclose information that is considered personal. Their views toward counseling may be influenced by the beliefs that the system is culturally insensitive, that there are few Spanish-speaking therapists, and that the "talking and listening" approach is geared more for mainstream Anglos than Latinos and is less effective than the assistance provided by folk healers. In addition, attitudes that stigmatize emotional problems and taboos against frank sexual discussions complicate the use of these interventions (Randall-David 1989). As a result, it may take much longer to engage the client.

The clinician has to allow time and be sensitive to cultural nuances that may appear in disguised forms. A desire for help, for example, may be handled covertly. The patient may be looking down, seemingly uninterested and uninvolved, while actually expecting the clinician to reach out and show her interest. How this is done is an important engagement issue. Offering coffee or a glass of water may be appropriate in the clinical setting, as it is considered a social grace and an example of *personalismo*. Establishing a personal relationship is very important in working with the Latino client. The clinical relationship, like other relationships, must adhere to the norms of dignity, politeness and respect, elements of *personalismo* (Dillard 1983). Latino clients will often describe an interaction with a clinician by stating, "He was like a good friend" or "She was like a cousin."

The clinician will find that beginning with a less confrontational approach and taking more time to develop trust and to establish a supportive relationship before discussing emotionally charged issues will be more effective with Latino clients. Strong listening skills are required in order to allow the client to express his or her individual experience of grief and loss. Although empathic listening is important in all clinical interventions, it is an expected cultural response in Latino culture. Strong expressions of empathy mark the clinician as an ally, someone on the client's side.

The role of clinician as champion and advocate is also an important one. Clinicians are expected to help their clients handle environmental stresses. Some Latino women, for example, are aware that their low socioeconomic condition places them at high risk for family stresses. They feel vulnerable and unable to negotiate the complexities of the American system of service delivery and public entitlements. They expect the clinician to help them understand how things are done in mainstream culture. Clinicians often have to educate their clients to the necessity of being on time for appointments and explaining when appointments must be broken. Latino clients may expect that the clinician will understand that other matters can take precedence over appointments.

Issues of disclosure of shameful information must be handled with great sensitivity and caution. If the clinician inadvertently shares information in a family meeting or with other health care providers or insists that the patient disclose information to the family, the clinician may in fact be placing the individual at risk. An example of this is the disclosure of the HIV status of a child, which may result in the rejection of the child by other family members, or disclosure of the bisexuality of a male family member, which could result in ostracism of that individual.

The clinician must also be very careful not to undermine the respect expected of children toward their parents. The parent may interpret any criticism of parenting behavior, particularly if it is done in front of the child, as a lack of respect. This holds true even if the child is sick. Sensitivity to this does not negate the necessity to encourage independence that is developmentally appropriate.

The clinician must also understand that it may take a long time for a grieving adult to cry in front of a family outsider. This should not be interpreted as a lack of feeling. While women are expected to be emotionally expressive, men, in general, are not. These gender role differences must be respected (Randall-David 1989). Time, empathic listening, and allowing the client to digress from the central issue are helpful. A more personal approach may be indicated, even sharing some personal information about the clinician's own experiences with sadness.

In helping children, it is important to understand the concrete ramifications of death for the child and to explain these to the child in an understandable fashion. For example, it is helpful to remind the child that he or she is not alone and that there are arrangements for caretaking and support, even if this is outside the extended family and involves the foster care system.

For children who have had little opportunity to talk about the experience, patience is required. Furman advocates an approach that educates the child to the concept of death, helping the child discuss other less dramatic experiences of death such as the death of a pet (Furman 1974). When developing young individuals are in latency or adolescent stages, Mishne (1983) suggests inquiring about their peer relationships during the assessment process. Friends and classmates may be included in group discussions.

The ability to conduct an interview in Spanish may be critical. Depending upon the degree of fluency or comfort in the use of English, some Latinos may be reluctant to be interviewed in English and may find it humiliating to discuss charged topics, fearing that they will not be fully understood (Garcia-Preto 1982). In particular, the use of Spanish may be comforting in times of grief.

Involvement of family members is paramount to reinforce support systems for the surviving child. Elderly family members should be included where feasible; women, as nurturers and family mediators, are critical participants. It is very important to help the family talk about the illness and to encourage open discussions within the family about future child custody arrangements, which may included legal procedures to ensure that parental choice of custody is protected. The realities of the situation must be presented in a way that will not overwhelm the family and will encourage the involvement of the child in planning for the future when it is appropriate.

The surviving parent must also be helped to cope so that he or she will remain emotionally available to the child. Family sessions are expected in Latino culture and attempts to resolve family conflicts can be encouraged within the session. It is expected that the clinician will respect existing family structures and hierarchies as well as belief systems such as those related to spiritualism.

Above all the clinician must be willing to understand the bicultural aspects that influence the family's functioning—values from Latino culture, values from Anglo culture. The clinician who attempts to understand the family's individual circumstances and struggles within the family's cultural context exhibits *respeto*, a highly valued attribute in Latino culture.

SUMMARY

For any child, death is an event of great magnitude, particularly when it occurs in the formative years. For the Latino orphan, as for all orphans, how death and the deprivations of life before death will be managed will depend greatly on the availability of family and community resources. The attitudes of their families will significantly influence how they cope and handle the dramatic and painful experiences of HIV-related death. It is important to help the child identify the cause of death; the cause is an immune deficiency, not a "bad" parent.

The richness of Latino culture, the significant value that children hold in the lives of both men and women, and the protective arms of the Latino family and community will help these surviving children to handle their sadness and grief. Strong religious faith, belief in an afterlife, and the hope that life after death will be better can offer additional comfort.

The professional community has a special responsibility to advocate for a supportive environment, to promote opportunities for communication within the family and the community, and to provide culturally sensitive clinical treatment. School personnel, health providers, and others who come in contact with children whose behavior shows symptoms that their emotional needs are not being met should be sensitive to the possibility that there may have been an AIDS death in the family. Children and their families should be referred to mental health services. There is, however, a lack of culturally sensitive mental health services. This is especially troublesome considering how difficult it is for many Latinos to go outside the family for help.

The orphans of the HIV/AIDS epidemic are generally children and adolescents whose parents have died young, most in their thirties and forties, a time when preparations should be for life and not for death. For these children there has often been little joy and much sorrow. Our mission must be to help families stay together when possible and, when not possible, to provide alternatives for children that provide nurturance and care.

REFERENCES

Caroff, P., and M. Mailick. 1985. "The Patient Has a Family: Reaffirming Social Work's Domain." *Social Work in Health Care* 10:17–35.

Centers for Disease Control. 1991. "Update: Acquired Immunodeficiency Syndrome—United States, 1981–1990." *Mobidity and Mortality Weekly Report* 40:358–369.

Centers for Disease Control and Prevention. 1993. *HIV/AIDS Surveillance*, Second Quarter Edition, 5(2).

Chau, K. 1991. "Social Work with Ethnic Minorities: Practice Issues and Potentials." *Journal of Multicultural Social Work* 1: 23–40.

Chu, Susan Y. 1993. Centers for Disease Control and Prevention, Division of HIV/AIDS. Personal correspondence, November 16.

Congress, E., and B. Lyon. 1992. "Cultural Differences in Health Beliefs: Implications for Social Work Practice in Health Settings." *Social Work in Health Care* 17:81–96.

Council on Scientific Affairs. 1991. "Hispanic Health in the United States." *Journal of the American Medical Association* 265:248–252.

Culturelinc Corporation. 1991. "Cultural Factors Among Hispanics: Perception and Prevention of HIV Infection." Albany AIDS Institute, New York State Department of Health.

Curtis, P. 1990. "The Consequences of Acculturation to Service Delivery and Research with Hispanic Families." *Child and Adolescent Social Work* 7:147–159.

de la Vega. 1990. "Consideration for Reaching the Latino Population With Sexuality and HIV/AIDS Information and Education." *SIECUS Report* 183:1–8.

Delgado, M., and D. Humm-Delgado. 1982. "Natural Support Systems: Source of Strength in Hispanic Communities." *Social Work* 27:85–89.

DeSpelder, L., and A. Strickland. 1987. *The Last Dance: Encountering Death and Dying*. Mountainview, CA: Mayfield.

Diaz, T., J. W. Buehler, K. G. Castro, and J. W. Ward. 1993. "AIDS Trends Among Hispanics in the United States." *American Journal of Public Health* 83:504–509.

Dillard, J. 1983. *Multicultural Counseling*. Chicago: Nelson-Hall.

Furman, E. 1974. *A Child's Parent Dies: Studies in Childhood Bereavement*. New Haven, CT: Yale University Press.

Garcia, Alejandro. 1991. "The Changing Demographic Face of Hispanics in the United States." In *Empowering Hispanic Families: A Critical Issue for the '90s*, ed. M. Sotomayor, 21–38. Milwaukee: Family Service of America.

Garcia-Preto, N. 1982. "Puerto Rican Families." In *Ethnicity and Family Therapy*, ed. M. McGoldrick, J. Pearce, and J. Giordano, 164–185. New York: The Guilford Press.

———. 1991. "Puerto Rican Families." In *Living Beyond Loss: Death in the Family*, ed. F. Walsh and M. McGoldrick, 142–194. New York: W. W. Norton.

Ghali, S. 1977. "Cultural Sensitivity and the Puerto Rican Client." *Social Casework* 55:100–110.

———. 1982. "Understanding Puerto Rican Traditions." *Social Work* 271:91–98.

Ginsberg, E. 1991. "Access to Health Care for Hispanics." *Journal of the American Medical Association* 265:238–241.

Gonzalez, G. 1991. "Hispanics in the Past Two Decades, Latinos in the Next Two: Hindsight and Foresight." In *Empowering Hispanic Families: A Critical Issue for the '90s*, ed. M. Sotomayer, 1–19. Milwaukee: Family Service of America.

Guendelman, S. 1990. "Developing Responsiveness to the Health Needs of Hispanic Children and Families." In *Social Work in Health Care*, ed. K. Davidson and S. Clarke, 713–730. New York: Haworth Press.

Harwood, A. 1981. *Ethnicity and Medical Care*. Cambridge, MA: Harvard University Press.

Ho, M. K. 1991. "Use of Ethnic-Sensitive Inventory ESI to Enhance Practitioner Skill with Minorities." *Journal of Multicultural Social Work* 1:57–68.

Jacobs, C., and D. Bowles, eds. 1988. *Ethnicity and Race: Critical Concepts in Social Work*. Washington, DC: National Association of Social Workers.

Kalish, R., and D. Reynolds. 1976. *Death and Ethnicity: A Psychocultural Study*. Los Angeles: The University of Southern California Press.

Latino Commission on AIDS. 1992. "Overview: Latinos and AIDS," Fact Sheet. New York City (December).

Leavitt, R., and M. Lutz. 1988. *Three Immigrant Groups in New York City: Dominicans, Haitians and Cambodians*. New York: Community Council of Greater New York.

Marin, B. 1990. "AIDS Prevention in Non-Puerto Rican Hispanics." In *AIDS and Intravenous Drug Use: Future Directions for Community Based Prevention Research*, ed. C. Leukefeld, R. J. Battjes, and Z. Amsel, 35–52. Washington, DC: US Government Printing Office, Publication No. 90–1627.

Michaels, D., and C. Levine. 1992. "Estimates of the Number of Motherless Youth Orphaned by AIDS in the United States." *Journal of the American Medical Association* 268(24):3456–3461.

Mishne, Judith. 1983. *Clinical Work with Children*. New York: Free Press.

Moore, J., and H. Panchon. 1985. *Hispanics in the United States*. Englewood Cliffs, NJ: Prentice-Hall.

National Commission on AIDS. 1992. *The Challenge of HIV/AIDS in Communities of Color*. Washington, DC: National Commission on AIDS.

New York City Department of Health. 1993. *AIDS Surveillance Update* (First Quarter).

New York City Department of Planning. 1990. *Demographic Profiles*.

Novello, A., P. Wise, and D. Kleinman. 1991. "Hispanic Health: Time for Data, Time for Action." *Journal of the American Medical Association* 265:253–255.

Randall-David, E. 1989. *Strategies for Working with Culturally Diverse Communities and Clients*. Washington, DC: Office of Maternal and Child Health, US Department of Health and Human Services, MCH #372004–03.

Rivera, E. 1990. "The Role of the Botanica Spiritualist and Santeria in the Latino Community Concerning HIV/AIDS." Report for the New York City Department of Health.

Rosenblatt, P. 1975. "Uses of Ethnography in Understanding Grief and Mourning." In *Bereavement, Its Psychosocial Aspects*, ed. B. Schoenberg, I. Gerber,

A. Weiner, A. Kutscher, D. Peretz, and A. Carr, 41–49. New York: Columbia University Press.

Sanchez, N. 1992. "Informal Adoption: The Extended Family and AIDS in the Latino Community." Presented to the Orphan Project, New York City, May 19.

Selik, R. M., S. Y. Chu, and J. W. Buehler. 1993. "HIV Infection as Leading Cause of Death Among Young Adults in U.S. Cities and States." *Journal of the American Medical Association* 263:1522–1525.

Soriano, F. 1991. "AIDS: A Challenge to Hispanics and Their Families." In *Empowering Hispanic Families: A Critical Issue for the '90s*, ed. M. Sotomayer, 59–74. Milwaukee: Family Service of America.

Stuntzner-Gibson, D. 1991. "Women and HIV Disease: An Emerging Crisis." *Social Work* 36:22–30.

US Department of Commerce, Bureau of the Census. 1989. *The Hispanic Population in the United States: March 1988*, Series P-20, No. 438. Washington, DC: US Department of Congress.

Wilfelt, A. 1983. *Helping Children Cope with Grief.* Muncie, IN: Accelerated Development.

Worden, J. W. 1991. *Grief Counseling and Grief Therapy: A Handbook for the Mental Health Practitioner.* New York: Springer.

7

Black American Communities: Coping with Death

Penelope Johnson-Moore
Lucretia J. Phillips

INTRODUCTION

When a person dies of AIDS, the process of grieving is very difficult for friends and families. This is largely because of widespread societal stigma and condemnation of the behaviors that are associated with the illness. The consequences of poverty, which plague the black community and are linked to the spread of AIDS, place additional hardships on blacks, who may be particularly hard hit with multiple losses and who may be bereft of economic and social structural supports to facilitate healthy mourning. Large numbers of black people may be blocked in their ability to work through various stages of grief and reach a state of adaptation where their losses can be resolved in a positive way. This lack of resolution increases blacks' vulnerability to physical and emotional depletion, commonly associated with abnormal or unsuccessful bereavement.

Data from the 1990 census show that black Americans have the highest rate of poverty in the United States: 31.9 percent as compared to 8.8 percent for white Americans. Moreover, 44.8 percent of black children live below the poverty line, compared with 15.9 percent of white youngsters. Social structures that maintain such dismal poverty for black Americans include a history of oppression, racism, and discrimination. The operation and strength of discriminatory practices are further manifested in the list of chronic problems confronting the black community such as poor education, unemployment, poor health care, and inadequate housing (Hacker 1992, 98–99).

In 1992, the highest annual rate of reported AIDS cases by race/ethnicity in the United States occurred among black Americans (52.2 per 100,000). By contrast, the rate among whites was 11.7 per 100,000 (CDC 1993a, 15). Although black Americans constitute only 12 percent of the population, 31 percent of reported AIDS cases as of July 1993 were among black Americans (CDC 1993b, 11). Afessa et al. (1992, 135) note that the incidence of AIDS among blacks is 34.9 per 100,000 compared with 9.6 per 100,000 population for whites. Black women account for 53 percent of all reported cases among women, and black children account for 55 percent of all reported pediatric cases (CDC 1993b, 9). The implications of these statistics are far-reaching when one considers the high death toll and the vast number of survivors left to grieve, whose grieving may be inhibited by stigma (Dane and Miller 1992).

How will the black American community cope with these deaths? What will sustain black Americans through these stigmatized losses? Trusting in the power of God will empower many black Americans to meet the pain of grieving losses resulting from AIDS. West (1991) identifies faith in God as a significant cultural feature that enables black people to cope with negative assaults. However, unique factors surrounding AIDS, such as stigma and secrecy, may force blacks to work harder to find within their own faith strategies for continuing to cope with both social structures that oppress and an illness that kills.

While this chapter will not focus on black people from other African and Caribbean cultures, it is important to note that Haitians as a subgroup of Caribbean blacks have been devastated by AIDS, as have American blacks born in the United States. However, special factors that influence Haitians' attitudes, beliefs, and ways of coping with AIDS death require a separate discussion. This chapter will emphasize broadening the understanding and meaning of various attitudes about AIDS-related deaths and barriers surrounding AIDS bereavement. It will also offer insights about the indigenous resources for facilitating successful bereavement in the black community.

RISK FACTORS AND ATTITUDES ABOUT AIDS IN THE BLACK COMMUNITY

Except for a few articles, there has been very little written specifically about the plight of significant others in the black community and their attempts to cope with AIDS deaths. Most articles identify the demographic profiles of various groups affected by AIDS, discuss risks associated with HIV transmission, and present various strategies for AIDS education and prevention. Several authors, such as Palacio and Weedy (1991), Wiener and Septimus (1991), and Grosz and Hopkins (1992), have documented broad systems issues and psychosocial considerations concerning minority children and families coping with AIDS. In the black community, factors generally linked to AIDS include poverty, homelessness, inadequate housing, fragmented social services, poor health care, and involvement with the welfare and legal systems that impact on families. These conditions provide a fertile ground for the sexual and drug-using behaviors that directly increase the risk of HIV transmission. AIDS all too frequently further undermines all structural supports available to the family and various significant others (Icard et al. 1992; Gray 1992; Lindan et al. 1990; Nyamathi and Shuler 1990; Honey 1988).

The sharing of injection equipment among drug users is the leading cause of HIV transmission in the black community (CDC 1993b, 7–8). Injecting drug use helps to maintain a cycle of oppression. Drug abusers are generally alienated from their families and support systems (Powell 1990; Cline 1990; Honey 1988; Pheifer and Houseman 1988). Dalton (1989, 217) eloquently captures the dilemma of drugs and AIDS in the black community.

On the one hand, blacks are scared to even admit the dimensions of the problem for fear that the whole black culture and its people will be viewed as junkies and as pathological. On the other, blacks desperately want to find solutions. Addicts prey on our neighborhoods, sell drugs to our children, steal our possessions, and rob us of hope. . . . We despise them because they hurt us and because they are us. . . . They are our sons and daughters, our sisters and brothers.

This dynamic tension increases the burden on significant others who are intolerant of the drug abuser's manipulative and, at times, abusive behaviors, as well as the financial hardship drug abuse places on the family.

Several authors discuss the issue of homophobia in the black community. Research investigating the attitudes of blacks toward homosexuality has identified several reasons why homosexuality is stigmatized by the black community. These include religious beliefs and the unavailability of many black men to become marriage partners and heads of households; this is largely because a disproportionate number of black men are in jail, suffer premature deaths due to disease and murder, and drop out of mainstream society because of mental illness, homelessness, and chronic unemployment (Ernst et al. 1991; Icard et al. 1992).

Dalton (1989, 215–217) offers a unique historical context for better understanding why black gay men may represent one of the most isolated groups of AIDS sufferers. Dalton hypothesizes that

homophobia has less to do with regulating sexual desire and affectional ties than with policing relations between the sexes. In this view, gay black men and lesbians are made to suffer because they are out of sync with a powerful cultural impulse to weaken black women and strengthen black men. . . . In other words, openly gay men and lesbians evoke hostility in part because they have come to symbolize the strong female and the weak male that slavery and a near century of societal Jim Crowism produced.

Nevertheless, many gay men and women have risen to prominence in the black community, for example, the late labor and civil rights leader Bayard Rustin. In fact, as Dalton says, "In practice black communities across the country have knowingly and sometimes fully embraced their gay members . . . [as long as] gay men and women have agreed . . . to downplay, if not hide, their sexual orientation."

According to Powell (1990), the greatest source of new HIV infections in the black community is heterosexual contacts between people who do not know they are infected. Wiener and Septimus (1991) indicate that issues of heterosexual transmission of HIV tend to cut across all social class and economic groups. These authors (p. 583) further state that "both in Black and Hispanic communities sexual practices reflect the established sex roles in which women are dominated by men and have fewer privileges. Women report that protection is used infrequently despite its necessity because they fear violence or rejection from their partners."

Nyamathi and Shuler's (1990, 1281) study of black women at risk for AIDS "revealed that Black women who practiced high risk activities experienced severely limiting environmental constraints that promoted a sense of powerlessness. These environmental constraints consisted of poverty, lack of adequate food and shelter, and a drug-rich environment in which there was no place to escape."

The mode of transmission seems to be important in determining how significant others in the black community respond to a person with AIDS. For example, the community may feel empathy for Arthur Ashe, a popular sports figure who contracted HIV from contaminated blood, or with Magic Johnson, whose positive HIV status is said to have resulted from heterosexual promiscuity, which is "positively" associated with masculinity. Unlike these two examples, however, a prostitute's or a bisexual man's HIV infections are viewed less compassionately because of their particular sexual routes of transmission. Additionally, these two cases may experience even less sympathy and support because they are seen as potentially infecting spouses and unborn children (Nyamathi and Shuler 1990).

BARRIERS TO EFFECTIVE BEREAVEMENT

Social stigma is a barrier to successful mourning. Biller and Rice (1990) indicate that losing a friend or lover to AIDS offers clues about one's own risk-taking behaviors, which can lead to a disruption in the traditional outlets of supportive grieving for survivors. Thus, survivors may be reluctant to attend a grief support group meeting and discuss their situation because of fear of being ostracized. Because blacks are fearful of racism and discrimination, many survivors may feel unwelcome in support groups organized by whites.

Bereavement overload associated with multiple losses makes it potentially difficult for black Americans to experience successful bereavement. Carmack (1992, 9) presents the concept of "bereavement overload" to describe the "overwhelming grief precipitated by the occurrence of multiple losses with little allowance for separate grieving time." Some black families may have several of their members living with the disease, or have family members who fall victim to violence or other illnesses.

In discussing the impact of AIDS on inner-city families, Dane and Miller (1992, 132) cite the prevalence of families' having to confront one crisis after another as an impediment to resolving grief. Not only do inner-city black and Latino families struggle against physical and economic difficulties, but they also struggle in their contacts with bureaucrats and professionals who are prone to attribute negative labels to them such as "disadvantaged," "impoverished," or "culturally deprived." Such a tendency among professionals inadvertently promotes a need for inner-city blacks to distance themselves from formal service providers in addressing various AIDS-related issues, including the issue of loss.

Denial as a mechanism of defense appears to be the major barrier to effective AIDS education and prevention in the black community. Denial also impedes mourning because families have difficulty acknowledging that a loved one is dying of AIDS, instead of cancer or some other less stigmatizing illness.

Aspects of denial and/or avoidance have also blocked the black church in moving quickly to confront the issue of AIDS. In a survey of 90 black Baptist ministers, which explored their attitudes about AIDS, Crawford et al. (1992, 309) found that "although most are aware that HIV infection poses a concern to their communities, most black ministers participating in the study did not perceive AIDS as being a significant threat." These findings support others who contend that the church's delay in responding to AIDS may be related to theological and ideological issues that condemn the "sin" of intravenous drug use and other high-risk behaviors. A shift, however, to thinking about AIDS as both human suffering and a medical problem may account for some readiness of churches to deliver AIDS-related services. This was particularly borne out in the survey of black Baptist ministers in that "80% of those surveyed indicated that they were willing to consider outreach and social service programming to be provided through their churches" (Crawford et al. 1992, 308).

Geographic and financial barriers present unique problems to some black families who may not have the financial resources to visit and participate in termination work with a loved one dying of AIDS. The account of a black woman whose brother died of AIDS demonstrates how successful mourning can take place, despite geographic distance, when financial hardship is not a factor.

Sue, the patient's sister, lived in Milwaukee with her family. John, the patient, lived in New York. Sue writes: "John kept secret from the family that he was gay until he was diagnosed with AIDS at age 35." From mid-1985 until his death in 1988, Sue visited her brother often in New York, where she met his homosexual friends. "I was treated with warmth and respect by his friends, but I associated AIDS with homosexuality. I had a lot of growing to do." Sue joined a support group, attended seminars in Milwaukee on homosexuality, and educated herself about AIDS. Besides traveling to New York, Sue spoke frequently with her brother on the telephone and lived in New York with him for most of his last 4 months.

A week before he died, John's insurance company forced him out of the hospital because of cost. Sue flew John to Milwaukee, where he died a week later in a nursing home. Sue indicated that she and John had both opportunity and courage to deal with multiple AIDS-related issues, including the shock of her brother's homosexuality, his shame and embarrassment at being found out through his illness, her anger about the illness and the lack of a cure, and his anger about his sickness and the gradual loss of control. In addition, both brother and sister experienced the range of emotions associated with AIDS—generalized anger, guilt, fear, task overload, and depression.

Despite the hardships, Sue remained guided by three factors: (1) her knowledge that her brother needed someone, which she refers to as a sister decision; (2) her belief that as a Christian she had a responsibility to embrace anyone who needed her (a faith decision); and (3) an overriding concern that her brother know that he was not alone.

Additional structural features that may create barriers to successful mourning behavior pertain to the negative impact of agency bureaucracies on the lives of black children placed in foster care as a result of abuse, neglect, inadequate familial supports and parents with AIDS. Institutions, which are governed by a plethora of legal systems and other bureaucratic structures, are unable to provide alternative care consistent with a child's psychological, emotional, and developmental needs. Not only is it difficult to deal with multiple agencies in planning and coordinating humane services, but most services are overwhelmed by the large numbers of people in need of them. Palacio and Weedy (1991, 570) indicate that in New York City alone, "since mid-1985 to mid-1989, the number of abuse and neglect cases filed in Family Court by HRA increased fourfold, from 2,792 cases to 11,300."

BEREAVEMENT ISSUES FOR CHILDREN SURVIVORS IN THE BLACK COMMUNITY

Since most children affected by AIDS are a product of high-risk environments, some discussion of cultural and class variables in child rearing practices in the black community is critical. Although no child may be immune to the negative impact of loss due to AIDS, black children who have not been constantly exposed to negative environmental assaults associated with high-risk environmental factors may have more available resources to meet the crisis of AIDS bereavement than do children whose lives are marked by constant chaos, crisis, and violence.

In a relatively stable environment, black Americans rely on their traditionally held beliefs concerning child rearing practices. An African proverb states, "It takes a village to raise a child." In general, the black American family believes that all children are special gifts to the parents. The broader community may believe that while children should "stay in their place," they should be treated with love and concern. In general, black families look forward to the joy in the birth of a child and give thanks to God that a child is born healthy, despite the social or economic status of the family unit (Peters 1981; Hines and Franklin-Boyd 1982; Logan et al. 1990).

Attitudes and expectations about children and child rearing patterns and practices are very much shaped by social class and life-style. However, despite class distinctions, the basic survival instincts of the black community have demanded that the family prepare children to deal with the forces of discrimination and racism in everyday American life, as well as how to meet their own biological, social, emotional, and psychological needs. Additional important cultural values have included teaching children to respect adults, protecting children, sharing of child rearing responsibility by both kin and nonkin adults, as well as handling discipline in a firm, no-nonsense manner.

Over time, however, traditional child rearing values have been undermined for poor blacks, particularly those trapped in inner cities by the constant struggle against poverty and the frequent exposure to drugs, guns, arson, and random violence (Parsons 1993, 1):

The inner city child witnesses injury, suffering, and death, and responds to these events with fear, grief, and often experience dramatic ruptures in their development. The list of psychological reactions is long and grim: hatred of self, profound loss of trust in the community and the world; tattered internalized moral values and ethics of caring, and a breaking down of the inner and outer sense of security and of reality. They are particularly vulnerable to traumatic stress illnesses, and to related behavioral and academic abnormalities.

In a discussion of the impact of AIDS on inner-city communities, Dane and Miller (1992, 132) focus on the difficulties of resolving grief in the face of a paucity of resources and the burden of dealing with multiple crises as a way of life. This environmental context poses a unique challenge to adult caregivers who may have traditional attitudes about protecting children and teaching them to become self-sufficient competent members of society. Unfortunately, the common occurrence of death in general and of AIDS-related deaths in particular forces surviving adults to push the developmental process so that children deal more directly with adult issues and possibly take on adult responsibilities. This situation is clearly documented in the sparse but growing literature on the impact of AIDS on children.

In a review of the literature, Grosz and Hopkins (1992, 45) cite the ramifications of HIV on the entire family, particularly children. Healthy brothers and sisters are left to bear the consequences of the illness on their family. While caregivers struggle to cope with the disease, these children must cope with the loss of their mothers, fathers, brothers, and sisters. Common themes emerging from the literature on brothers and sisters show them to be at risk as a result of their experience of significant stress. Stress-provoking conditions may include 1) being kept uninformed about the AIDS illness in the family; 2) children's avoidance of asking questions to protect their parents, 3) participation in the care of an ill parent, which de-emphasizes care and attention to the child's own needs, 4) anxieties children may have about their own health status, and 5) anxieties about their future when the parent dies. These authors (Grosz and Hopkins 1992, 45) conclude that

the long-term psychological implications for children survivors of AIDS deaths are enormous. Facing the fear of the gradual deterioration and eventual death of a beloved parent causes ongoing and vast psychological pressure and stress. Brothers and sisters will need to rebuild their lives, learn to trust, feel wanted, and become reincorporated into new families before they can overcome such overwhelming losses.

In a recent study of 38 inner-city children conducted by Schilling et al. (1992, 405-419), it was noted that socioeconomic stress may interact with the mourning process, making it more difficult for poor children to mourn. Dane and Miller (1992) make a similar observation in their work with inner-city families and advocate flexibility in existing models of bereavement to take into account the social and cultural variables and the unique customs, concerns, and responses of inner-city residents to loss and grief. A psychodynamic understanding of challenges facing the black inner-city child also requires a multilevel view of developmental, ecological, and social class perspectives that can offer clues about their issues and needs concerning bereavement.

THE BLACK CHURCH, RELIGION, AND AIDS

Each cultural group has its own belief system regarding good and evil spirits, healing practices, life after death, and death-related rituals or behavioral styles. When reviewing the literature on the black American family, cultural variables usually include references to the importance of the family group, particularly extended family, and the role of religion in the group's survival, coping, and adaptation.

The importance of the black church and religion in the lives of black people has been succinctly summarized by Dane and Miller (1992, 148):

The church has been a stabilizing force in family and community life since slavery. . . . The church has been and continues to be the context in which many secular institutions developed. It is the original African American self-help institution and a safe place for emotional release. The church provides spiritual leadership and emotional and financial supports. Participants are offered opportunities for educational advancement, socialization and participation in social change activities. This institution represents, for active participants, a viable extended family.

Since slavery, the church has also represented a place where one's sense of justice and right is experienced, and where one's faith and endurance are supported. Kilgoe's (1992, 5–7) documentation of the origins of the black church emphasizes the need for a separate institution of worship based on the survival needs of black Americans: "The black church offered the hope of freedom to slaves during their worship experiences and prayer services. They became confident that the same God of Abraham, Isaac, and Jacob was also the God of Moses who led the Israelites out of bondage in Egypt, and that the same God could deliver them from slavery."

Kilgoe (1992) concurs with other authors who confine their definition of the black church to Methodist, Baptist, and Pentecostal groups rather than other mainline religious denominations or sects that were crafted by oppressors in the white church. "The practicing religion of churches started by blacks is a theology of survival. It is also a carrier of the black folk culture. The practicing religion of the white church, with certain exceptions, has been American culture and racism."

Kilgoe (1992) also quotes Emmanuel McCall, who summarizes the separatist aims of black churches. "For any cultural expression of faith to have validity and utility, the people must establish themselves in their own vernacular. Black denominationalism was and continues to represent a movement in that direction."

Lincoln and Mamiya (1990) explored the religious dimensions of the black church and proposed that a "dialectical model" of analysis be employed to understand the unique functioning of the church in the black community. The dialectical model examines the dynamic interplay among black American history, culture, and religion as a strategy of survival within the present-day context of social conditions, including the situation of the church's leadership and membership at any given time. The particular orientation of a given church regardless of its denomination may deal with one set of tensions versus another, depending on congregational needs. Thus, a clear differentiation between church and state, as one may find in white church denominations, may be less likely in black churches.

Hill (1971) not only concurs with various authors' (Lincoln and Mamiya 1990; Dillard 1993, 146; Kilgoe 1992; Dane and Miller 1992) assessment of the centrality of the church's role in the black community, but addresses the way in which religion helps to shape the worldview of blacks as it relates to life and death. He asserts that racism and intergroup and intragroup violence have forced black Americans to confront and deal with death from both natural and unnatural causes continuously.

Religion and spirituality can give a perspective to the profound problems of social reality, in that it provides an opportunity for survival. The ability to cope with multiple losses has to involve, among other things, finding avenues of renewal and ways of keeping faith and having hope that things will get better. For black Americans, the ability to cope with so many societal assaults is linked with faith, the belief that "God is good and generous," and that "trusting in the Lord" will get one through day by day. As true of other cultural groups, the religious attitudes, death rituals, resources for support, and ways of expressing grief serve as coping strategies and facilitate the resolution of grief by the bereaved (York and Stichler 1985, 125).

Worden (1982) clearly indicates that affective expression is important to the mourning process, as the bereaved need to have permission to express feelings. When this is not encouraged, adequate resolution of grief may not be accomplished.

Given the broad structural barriers to overcoming oppression in American society and to enfranchising grieving in the black community, the question to be addressed is, How does a community of people who are largely bereft of resources organize a meaningful response to AIDS illness? West (1991, 223) points to

the genius of black foremothers and forefathers who equipped black folk with cultural armor to beat back the demons of hopelessness, meaninglessness, and lovelessness. These buffers consisted of cultural structures of meaning and feeling that created and sustained communities. This armor constituted ways of life and struggle that embodied values of service and sacrifice, love and care, discipline and excellence that nurtured traditions for black surviving and thriving under usually adverse new world conditions. These traditions consist primarily of black religious and civic institutions that sustained familial and communal networks of support.

If we accept these concepts, then it is important to examine a unique aspect of the black community: its Christian belief system and the enfranchised grieving permitted in the church service rituals, no matter what the cause of death or how heavy the burden. Worship through prayer, gospel, and song are some of the powerful aspects of church service practices. General Sunday worship ritual, Wednesday night prayer meeting, Bible study and annual revival meetings provide cathartic opportunities. One can find ways through these rituals to express profound grief about one's loss and the multiple losses experienced in a family, among friends, and in the immediate community. Even if an individual is marginal to the formal church, there is always someone in the community who attends church and who will pray for the bereaved. A colleague who is part of a prayer line for her church talks about the increased number of calls from people with AIDS who are dying. They call asking for "God's mercy," for "salvation," and for "forgiveness." She is one of more than twenty on the prayer line who will offer a prayer for the caller.

The morning prayer at Sunday worship is often a general prayer giving thanks for life, seeking guidance, and asking that God be with those who are in need (the sick, bereaved, those in crisis, and so on). "Lord, have mercy" is a much-used phrase by many black Americans, as is "God knows how much you can bear," which suggests one will surely get through the pain of loss, crisis, or any other extraordinary event(s).

Henderson and Primeaux (1981, 21) refer to Kaplan, who succintly describes the powerful aspects of the revival meeting:

Enter a (Protestant) revival and one witnesses yelling, wailing, crying, and talking in tongues. During the sermon, the audience participates in frequent yelling and prancing about. The songs are sung with the fullest possible emotional commitment, often with tears. After singing, the preacher and the congregation often break into what is called "talking in tongues," which is an expression of whatever comes to mind in a seemingly disorderly way with unique words, which are seen as presumably the Divine speaking through man. (Kaplan 1965, 134–136)

Along the continuum—from speaking in tongues to less overt forms of expression—the revival represents a time for coming together, a time of support, and a time for asking forgiveness and praying for self and others. These rituals help to reframe a negative experience, such as a death, through religious teaching and reaffirmation of faith. When all else fails, one can go to the altar and hand his/her troubles over to the Lord—"Let go, Let God."

FUNERAL RITUALS IN THE BLACK CHURCH

Ludwig (1989, 178) notes, "Death is considered by Christians as a passage to the life promised and won by Christ, so death rituals combine the sense of loss and sadness with the mood of joy and confidence . . . and a funeral is a time to commend the departed one to the company of 'Saints' awaiting the resurrection and eternal life in heaven." He goes on to say that a funeral is a time to reflect on the brevity of life and the destiny that awaits all. It is a time to renew hope and confidence in God's mercy and promises.

The funeral ritual is a very important ceremony in the black community. The funeral may be elaborate or simple, but the custom is very similar. The ceremony includes prayers, songs, viewing of the body, and eulogy by the minister. Children usually do not attend the wake, but it is expected that, depending upon their age, they will attend the funeral of their parent and go to the grave for the burial.

Kalish and Reynolds (1976 , 110) point out the importance of funerals for blacks: "When a society treats a people as objects, accords them only minimal respect, and simultaneously blocks the channel by which respect can be achieved, the result is, predictably, a people who desperately seek ways to confirm some sense of self-worth and positive self identity."

AIDS-related deaths may present a dilemma for those charged with eulogizing the deceased. The following case example illustrates some issues related to funeral planning for someone who died of AIDS. This case points out practical problems faced by the family in making funeral arrangements and highlights aspects of denial that make it more difficult for significant others to use the prescribed time of mourning allowed by the funeral ceremony effectively.

Mrs. G's daughter, D, died of an AIDS-related complication. She had been a longtime drug abuser and was often estranged from her family. Mrs. G and her mother have been responsible for D's children, ages 3, 7, and 9. Following the resolution of the "battle" about how ready the 7- and 9-year-old were to handle the wake and funeral (it was determined early on that the 3-year-old would not attend the wake or funeral), the next "battle" was the location of the funeral. Mrs. G's mother insisted that the funeral take place in a church, even though Mrs. G did not think it a good idea, since D did not belong to the church. In addition, D was said to have been "a very long way from God's way." Mrs. G finally gave in, and there was a church service funeral. While Mrs. G felt relieved about the end of her daughter's suffering, she also felt a tremendous sense of what she called "spiritual peace."

The church service did give some dignity to her daughter in death, even though she had not led a dignified life. No one talked about the cause of D's death, and after the burial, friends and family did what is always done after funerals: They carried food and drinks to Mrs. G's home, supported her, cried when she cried, and talked throughout the evening about "the old times."

The funeral ritual served a vital function for the family, in that it could symbolically purge the "sin" of AIDS and provide a sense of dignity to the family. It provided a mechanism for bringing together family and friends of the deceased to begin to come to terms with the deceased's life-style and stigmatized illness. The ritual also afforded time to pray for things to be better for D in the "hereafter." All of the children were able to participate in the mourning process; they talked about how they felt when their mother was ill. Discussion focused on the service, the songs and the many "pretty flowers"—the things that helped the children to normalize the death and discuss it without shame. From her two older sisters, the 3-year-old heard a full description of the funeral, but she was not told the cause of her mother's death. Their friends did not ask about the cause of death; many of them have also lost a parent from AIDS or violent death. Although the shame, anger, and embarrassment related to an AIDS death need to be more openly discussed, the family did take the first step in that direction through the wake, funeral, burial, and the sharing that continued after the burial. At a later time, the family may be able to take advantage of a support group or become involved with clinical services to continue working through issues of grief and bereavement.

THE ROLE OF THE FUNERAL DIRECTOR

The funeral director is a critical actor in the funeral ritual. In the black community, funeral directors are distinguished as special community folk along with ministers, teachers, physicians, and other professionals. The use of a particular mortician and his services is as much a part of the funeral planning as is the ritual itself. Most often the director has planned with the family over many years and buried a number of family members.

As an integral part of the community and family systems, the mortician can greatly influence the family's decisions through his beliefs and attitudes. The mortician's role is particularly important as he has the power either to block or to enable the bereavement work of the family. When the relationship between funeral director and family is strong and spans a long period, he understands the customs as well as the religious and cultural values of the family and is therefore more likely to be supportive. This role very much parallels that of the minister.

However, just as AIDS-related deaths pose a dilemma to ministers and other helping professionals, so too has it affected the special relationship between families and morticians. Funeral directors have expressed fears about contact with the deceased's bodily fluids, personal attitudes about the behaviors related to HIV transmission, the increasing number of deaths from AIDS, and the almost daily need to deal with this particular type of death. Additionally, the "look" of the body (loss of weight, discoloration of the skin, loss of teeth and hair) presents problems for directors who are concerned about the proper preparation of the body. Some have encouraged cremation, a method of disposition of the body rarely utilized by black families.

Contrary to cultural tradition, some black families may be urged to have a closed casket. This interferes with the family custom of "sitting" with the body at the wake before the funeral, thus blocking the family's ability to maximize the opportunity of the funeral to work toward a resolution of grief. Although children may be protected from direct involvement with the mortician, the impact on the family will be experienced. Cremation and closed coffins, in particular, will raise questions by children, as well as others, that the adult survivors may feel too ill prepared or too guilty to answer.

Rando (1984, 196) highlights the power and symbolism of the funeral director. "The very same limousines that carry the families of the deceased to the cemetery are also those that carry families to their weddings." This association is particularly important for black families whose dependence on the mortician for a broad array of services may blur appropriate boundaries and skew critical issues of significance to families in planning the funeral of a loved one who has died of AIDS.

SERVICE DELIVERY

Rogler et al. (1983) developed a conceptual framework regarding service delivery systems and the underutilization of social services by Puerto Rican families, which is applicable to black families as well. The barrier and alternate resource theories he suggests are useful in understanding patterns of underutilization. The barrier theory, as opposed to "blaming the victim," looks at the service delivery system as lacking a true responsiveness to clients' needs. In the alternate resource theory, families make use of familiar social organizations within their culture to deal with their problems. For black families, the use of the extended family and reliance on Christian faith and religious organizations have traditionally been regarded as alternative resources to government or mainstream social services. An example of the integration of religion in developing an alternative resource for black families dealing with AIDS loss is the Mother's Love Support Group in Brooklyn, New York:

The group was founded by Mother Pearson, who has lost two sons to AIDS within the past 5 ½ years. The impetus to start a support group came in February 1988, following the death of her 30–year-old son whom the family cared for at home for 7 months prior to death. Although Mother Pearson had lost another son who had contracted HIV through injecting drug abuse, she states, "I did not initially come forth regarding this son because I wanted to protect my grandchildren and his family, who were not yet ready to deal with this issue in the public eye."

Initially, Mother Pearson contacted the Gay Men's Health Crisis (GMHC), where her son had a "buddy" who visited him once a week during his illness. After spending some time in volunteer activities, Mother Pearson became involved with the Brooklyn AIDS Task Force (BATF), where she was encouraged to tell her story to others. The BATF put Mother Pearson in touch with a mothers' group in Manhattan. After learning how the group operated, Mother Pearson was ready to form her own support group. "I told Fran (the Manhattan Group leader) that I'd like to start a similar group in Brooklyn in the minority community. Her group was geared mostly towards middle class whites, and I knew we needed help amongst ourselves. . . .

"We started out very slowly, meeting together behind closed doors, lifting each other up. We cry sometimes; we tell each other about the pain that we had this week, or last. In our group, we pray out loud, or if you don't want to pray out loud, you can meditate. But it's all the same language. Some mothers who come in are not spiritually inclined. But on this trail that we walk, we have nobody else to talk to but God Almighty. And He stands firm and He holds us up. Mothers go through some very lonely hours."

Mother Pearson subsequently left the Brooklyn AIDS Task Force in order to reach a broader span of people in her own community. The group has expanded to include not only families who have experienced loss, but also young mothers living with HIV/AIDS. In the group, they receive support around their parenting roles and their efforts to prepare their children for the eventuality of death.

The Mother's Love Support Group was offered space in Mother Pearson's church, and in 1990 the group received a grant from the Citizen's Committee for New York City. Modest grant funds and private contributions help the group maintain a telephone hotline for people with AIDS and their significant others and cover basic operating costs.

In discussing some of the therapeutic aspects of the group, Mother Pearson indicates that group members are challenged to confront issues of denial, discuss their feelings of isolation, and share the pain of loss. New members are also challenged to reconnect with their own faith, since ultimately the belief is that dependence on God is the only way to go through the pain of losing a child, especially when parents may have to bury more than one child, as Mother Pearson has. Faith is believed to help parents deal with their problems through open, honest communication in the group. Each group ends with holding hands and prayer.

The Mother's Love Support Group models several key principles of the alternate resource theory that are instructive for other helping professionals who want to broaden AIDS bereavement services in the black community. It emphasizes the importance of offering services in the church and in the locations where the people coping with or caring for someone with AIDS live. The church helps to diminish the burden of getting needed help before, during, and after a death. The church is also a natural link to the minister. Thomas and Dansby (1985) indicate that black families are just as likely to go to their ministers as they are to a social agency. The church is the central meeting place in the community and a place where black people invest much time, money, and commitment to providing a range of social services (i.e., recreation, senior citizen housing, preschool programs, and feeding the homeless). It represents a natural arena for bolstering self-help initiatives and expanding community outreach and prevention programs.

The Brooklyn AIDS Task Force and GMHC were excellent models of professional providers and informal caregivers working collaboratively to enlarge services to vulnerable populations. These organizations offered practical guidance, advice, and support to help Mother Pearson get her own group off the ground. Members of the group can now help one another through sharing, support, and education. As is generally true of self-help groups, members help to combat the isolation of loss, family problems, and stigma.

In a broader context, the Mother's Love group also links informal caregivers to larger communities of caregivers, as well as to formal service providers. Mother Pearson has become both a local and a national spokesperson on the impact of AIDS on the family. She and her support group members have spoken to high school students about AIDS education and prevention. She has given presentations to groups in Sioux City, Iowa, Boston, and Atlanta. She has spoken to lay people, ecumenical groups, and politicians.

Finally, the Mother's Love Support Group demonstrates how community programs can become more integrated in the black community. Taylor et al. (1989) advocate increased outreach efforts, such as home visiting, as an important component of the alternate resource model. Home visiting ensures timely delivery of services and can minimize certain obvious barriers to securing help. Mother Pearson articulates this beautifully when she says, "When things get so rough that a mother can't come to meetings, or she's stuck at the hospital, we have taken the meetings to her, to hold her up during his time, because it's a lonely trail." Home visiting programs may identify those who are alone in their grief. Community programs that work in concert with already established institutions probably have the potential for reaping the best benefits. For example, a multiservice center located in a church, staffed by professionals and paraprofessionals or community residents, with a well-publicized telephone hotline in an accessible location may even diminish the need for home visiting.

In light of the rapidly growing number of black children in need of services, interventions in the school setting can play a critical role in targeting the bereavement needs of children and adolescents. The school is a natural link to the black community and is a valuable resource for providing direct clinical and preventive services to children and families experiencing AIDS losses. Accessibility of services in schools may also diminish caregivers' resistance to seeking bereavement help for children and, therefore, may combat a tendency to disenfranchise their grief process.

A model of school intervention operates in the New York City school system, where the Board of Education, the New York City Department of Mental Health, Mental Retardation and Alcoholism Services, and various mental health agencies have formed a partnership to offer clinical and preventive mental health services in designated schools. Although these programs focus broadly on the psychological, behavioral, and adjustment needs of children, they also reach many children affected by AIDS. Bereavement groups for children, surviving grandparents, foster parents, and other caregivers may be less stigmatizing and more effective when conducted within the school rather than in settings outside the immediate community.

SUMMARY AND RECOMMENDATIONS

This chapter has elucidated some unique factors to be considered in understanding AIDS-related death and bereavement in the black community. In order to broaden bereavement services and to facilitate successful grieving, these authors believe that it is important to work with the strengths of the black community in the context of their faith and belief system. Therefore, we wish to make the following recommendations:

1. Mental health professionals need to possess good clinical assessment skills that help them to determine the extent to which grief reactions are normal or abnormal within the cultural context of black people. Requisite skills would need to include a multilevel integrated assessment of the person in environment configuration. Particular attention should be given to the strengths of black families as well as to race, culture, life stressors and poverty as they affect black people's overall functioning and their cultural response to AIDS-related illness and death.

2. Mental health professionals should be knowledgeable about HIV infection and AIDS in order to help adult caregivers to increase their knowledge of the disease, its course of illness, and the special concerns related to secrecy, confidentiality and legal issues.

3. Clinicians need a sound knowledge base concerning bereavement interventions and the stages of grieving in order to normalize the bereavement experiences of black families and to educate families about the various stages of grief.

4. Mental health professionals must strive to develop culturally sensitive, child-centered interventions that allow children affected by HIV/AIDS to be children. Attention to children's developmental needs within the context of a therapeutic alliance can facilitate their ability to work through sadness, grief, loss, and other emotions associated with bereavement.

5. Mental health professionals should be knowledgeable about the alternate resource model of intervention with people of color and possess the competence to assist in facilitating the development of self-help programs in the community.

6. Mental health professionals need to develop collaborative relationships with informal service providers and various health, mental health, and social service providers in order to improve coordination and integration of a broad spectrum of services for families presenting a range of needs.

7. Service providers should be knowledgeable about the function of religion in the lives of black people and broaden their assessment tools to determine the value of promoting linkages with churches and ministers as a source of help and informal support.

NOTE

We want to express our appreciation to the many colleagues who reviewed our material. In particular, we are grateful to Karen Hopkins, M.D., the Reverend Dr. Tyrone E. Kilgoe, and Mildred "Mother" Pearson for their special contributions in the development of the chapter.

REFERENCES

Afessa, Bekele, William Green Greaves, Lateef Olopoenia, Robert Delapenha, Carl Saxinger, and Frederick Winston. 1992. "Autopsy Findings in HIV-Infected Inner City Patients." *Journal of Acquired Immune Deficiency Syndromes* 5:132–136.

Biller, Ray, and Susan Rice. 1990. "Experiencing Multiple Loss of Persons with AIDS: Grief and Bereavement Issues." *Health and Social Work* 15:283–290.

Carmack, Betty J. 1992. "Balancing Engagement/Detachment in AIDS-related Multiple Losses." *Image: Journal of Nursing Scholarship* 24:9–14.

Centers for Disease Control and Prevention. 1993a. *HIV/AIDS Surveillance Report* (U.S. AIDS cases reported through December 1992, issued February 1993), Year-End Edition.

———. 1993b. *HIV/AIDS Surveillance Report*, Second Quarter Edition, 5(2).

Cline, Dorothy Jean. 1990. "The Psychosocial Impact of HIV Infection: What Clinicians Can Do to Help." *Journal of the American Academy of Dermatology* 22:1299–1302.

Cooley, Mary E. 1992. "Bereavement Care: A Role for Nurses." *Cancer Nursing* 15:125–129.

Crawford, Isiaah, Kevin W. Allison, W. LaVome Robinson, Donna Hughes, and Maria Samaryk. 1992. "Attitudes of African American Baptist Ministers Toward AIDS." *Journal of Community Psychology* 20:304–307.

Dalton, Harlon L. 1989. " AIDS in Blackface." *Daedalus* 118:205–227.

Dane, Barbara O., and Samuel O. Miller. 1992. "Intervening with Inner-City Survivors of AIDS." In *AIDS: Intervening with Hidden Grievers*. Westport, CT: Auburn House.

Dillard, John M. 1993. *Multicultural Counseling*. Chicago: Nelson-Hall.

Doka, Kenneth J., ed. 1989. *Disenfranchised Grief: Recognizing Hidden Sorrow*. Lexington, MA: Lexington Books.

Ellis, Richard R. 1990. "Young Children: Disenfranchised Grievers." In *Disenfranchised Grief: Recognizing Hidden Sorrow*, ed. K. J. Doka. Lexington, MA: Lexington Books.

Ernst, Frederick A., Rupert A. Francis, Harold Nevels, and Carol Lemeh. 1991. "Condemnation of Homosexuality in the Black Community: A Gender Specific Phenomenon?" *Archives of Sexual Behavior* 20:579–585.

Fawzy, I., Nancy Fawzy, and Robert O. Pasnau. 1991. "Bereavement in AIDS." *Psychiatric Medicine* 9:469–482.

Gibbs, Jewelle Taylor, and Larke Nahme Huang. 1989. *Children of Color*. San Francisco: Jossey-Bass.

Gray, Gloria A. 1992. "Facing Terminal Illness in Children with AIDS: Developing a Philosophy of Care for Patients, Families and Caregivers." *Home Healthcare Nurse* 10:40–42.

Grosz, Jenny, and Karen Hopkins. 1992. "Family Circumstances Affecting Caregivers and Brothers and Sisters." In *HIV Infection and Developmental Disabilities*, ed. A. C. Crocker, H. J. Cohen, and T. A. Kastner. Baltimore: Paul H. Brookes.

Hacker, Andrew. 1992. *Two Nations, Black and White, Separate, Hostile, Unequal*. New York: Charles Scribner's Sons.

Henderson, George, and Martha Primeaux, eds. 1981. *Transcultural Health Care*. Menlo Park, CA: Addison-Wesley.

Hill, Robert B. 1971. *The Strengths of Black Families*. New York: National Urban League, Inc.

———. 1987. "Building the Future of the Black Family." *American Vision* 2:16–25.

Hines, Paulette M., and Nancy Franklin-Boyd. 1982. "Black Families." In *Ethnicity and Family Therapy*, ed. M. McGoldrick, J. K. Pearce, J. Giordano, 85–107. New York: Guilford Press.

Honey, Ellen. 1988. "AIDS and the Inner City: Critical Issues." *Social Casework: Journal of Contempory Social Work* 69:365–370.

Icard, Larry D., Robert F. Schilling, Nabila El-Bassel, and Dale Young. 1992. "Preventing AIDS Among Black Gay Men and Heterosexual Male Intravenous Drug Users." *Social Work* 37:440–445.

Jacob, John E. 1991. "Black America, 1990: An Overview." In *The State of Black America*, National Urban League, 1–8. New York: National Urban League.

———. 1992. "Black America, 1991: An Overview." In *The State of Black America*, National Urban League, 1–9. New York: National Urban League.

Kalish, R. A., and D. K. Reynolds. 1976. *Death and Ethnicity: A Psychocultural Study*. Los Angeles: University of Sothern California Press.

Kaplan, B. H. 1965. "The Structure of Adaptive Sentiments in a Lower Class Religious Group in Appalachia." *Journal of Social Issues* 21:134–135.

Kastenbaum, Robert J. 1991. *Death, Society, and Human Experience*, 4th ed. New York: Merrill.

Kilgoe, Tyrone E. 1992. "Picking up the Pieces: Rebuilding an African American Baptist Church After Congregational Separation." Doctor of Ministry Dissertation, United Theological Seminary, Philadelphia.

Lincoln, Eric C., and Lawrence H. Mamiya. 1990. *The Black Church in the African American Experience*. Durham, NC: Duke University Press.

Lindan, Christina P., Norman Hearst, James A. Singleton, Alan I. Trachtenberg, Noleen M. Riordan, Diane A. Tokagowa, and George S. Chu. 1990. "Underreporting of Minority AIDS Deaths in San Francisco Bay Area, 1985–86." *Public Health Reports* 105:400–404.

Logan, Sadye, Edith M. Freeman, and Ruth G. McRoy. 1990. *Social Work Practice with Black Families: A Culturally Specific Perspective*. New York: Longman.

Ludwig, Theodore M. 1989. *The Sacred Paths: Understanding the Religions of the World*. New York: Macmillan.

Nichols, E. K. 1989. "Mobilizing Against AIDS: The Unfinished Story of a Virus," rev. ed. Washington DC: National Academy of Sciences.

Nyamathi, Adeline, and Pam Shuler. 1990. "Focus Group Interview: A Research Technique for Informed Nursing Practice." *Journal of Advanced Nursing* 15:1281–1288.

Palacio, Christina, and Chris Weedy. 1991. "Treatment Issues Regarding Children in Foster Care." In *Pediatric AIDS: The Challenge of HIV Infection in Infants, Children and Adolescents*, ed. P. A. Pizzo and C. M. Wilfert. Baltimore: Williams & Wilkins.

Parson, Erwin Randolph. 1993. "Inner City Children of Traumatic Stress Response Syndrome M-VTS and Therapists' Response." In *Countertransference in the*

Treatment of Post-Traumatic Stress Disorder, ed. John P. Wilson and Jacob Lundy. New York: Guildford Press.

Pearson, Mildred. 1990. "Mother Pearson of Mother's Love." *The Body Positive* 3(4):19–22.

Peters, Marie F. 1981. "Parenting in Black Families with Young Children: A Historical Perspective." In *Black Families*, ed. H. P. McAdoo. Newbury Park, CA: Sage.

Pheifer, William G., and Clare Houseman. 1988. "Bereavement and AIDS: A Framework for Intervention." *Journal of Psychosocial Nursing* 26:21–26.

Powell, Dorothy L. 1990. "Health Care Crisis in the Black Community: Challenges, Prospects, and the Black Nurse." *Journal National Black Nurses Association* 51:3–10.

Rando, Therese A. 1984. *Grief, Dying and Death, Clinical Interventions for Caregivers.* Champaign, IL: Research Press.

Rogler, Lloyd, Rosemary Cooney, Guiseppe Constantino, Brian Earley, Beth Grossman, Douglas Gurak, Robert Malgady, and Orland. Rodriquez. 1983. *A Conceptual Framework for Mental Health Research on Hispanic Populations.* New York: Hispanic Research Center.

Schilling, Robert, N. Koh, Robert Abromovitz, and Louisa Gilbert. 1992. "Bereavement Groups for Inner-City Children." *Research on Social Work Practice* 23:405–419.

Swinton, David H. 1991. "The Economic Status of African Americans: Permanent Poverty and Inequality." In *The State of Black America 1991*, National Urban League, 22–75. New York: National Urban League.

———. 1992. "The Economic Status of African Americans: Limited Ownership and Persistent Inequality." In *The State of Black America 1992*, National Urban League, 61–117. New York: National Urban League.

Taylor, Robert J., Harold W. Neighbors, and Clifford L. Broman. 1989. "Evaluation by Black Americans of the Social Service Encounter During a Serious Personal Problem." *Social Work* 34:205–211.

Thomas, Michele B., and Pearl G. Dansby. 1985. "Black Clients: Family Structures, Therapeutic Issues, and Strengths." *Psychotherapy* 22(2S):398–407.

West, Cornel. 1991. "Nihilism in Black America. A Danger That Corrodes from Within." *Dissent* 3:221–226.

Wiener, Lori, and Anita Septimus. 1991 "Psychosocial Consideration and Support for the Child and Family." *Pediatric AIDS: The Challenge of HIV Infection in Infants, Children and Adolescents*, ed. P. A. Pizzo and C. M. Wilfert. Baltimore: Williams & Wilkins.

Worden, J. William. 1982. *Grief Counseling and Grief Therapy.* New York: Springer.

Wright, Gloria. 1991. "The People Touched by AIDS." *The Milwaukee Journal Magazine* (27 October).

York, Colette, R., and Jaynelle F. Stichler. 1985. "Cultural Grief Expressions Following Infant Death." *Family Strategies* 4:120–127.

8
Bereavement and the New Guardians

Gary R. Anderson

Almost from the very first reported cases of women with AIDS, society has been faced with the specter of children being orphaned by the death of one or both parents to the disease. Most of these women have been of childbearing age, and from 20 to 30 percent of their children born after they became HIV-infected will be HIV-infected themselves. A study of the first 60 pediatric HIV cases in specialized foster care in New York City found that the majority of mothers were seriously ill with HIV-related illnesses or unavailable; almost all the biological fathers were dead, were very ill, had unknown whereabouts or identities, or were in prison (Anderson and Gurdin unpublished).

Other mothers became HIV-infected after their children were born. Although these children are not HIV-infected, their primary caregivers have been faced with multiple obstacles to caring for themselves and their families. The result of this devastation to the primary, traditional caretakers of children—their biological parents—has been frequent reliance on other family structures. These structures include living with relatives, kinship foster care, family foster care, independent group living, and adoptive families. Each structure, while providing necessary shelter and support, may also pose complications for children's grieving processes. These arrangements raise clinical and legal issues as well as complications for the bereavement process.

RELATIVES AND KINSHIP CARE

Bowlby describes the absolute importance of attachment—the connection between an infant or child and a loving caregiver:

[W]hat is believed to be essential for mental health is that the infant and young child should experience a warm, intimate, and continuous relationship with his mother (or permanent mother-substitute) in which both find satisfaction and enjoyment. (Bowlby 1967, 11)

In addition to acknowledging the importance of attachment, one must also consider the harmful effects of certain types of deprivations, including separation from the mother. The deprivation of maternal care results in varying degrees of acute anxiety, an excessive need for love, and strong feelings of revenge. Guilt and depression can result from these feelings. A child's grieving is painful and potentially harmful to his or her future psychological and social development. This deprivation can be attributed to disturbances in the mother-child relationship as well as to their physical separation.

The guiding principle of Bowlby's work is that the "right place for a child is in his own home" (p. 109). Helping a parent to care for his or her child and emphasizing attachment between parent and child are Bowlby's main concerns.

In the early 1980s there were few services for women with HIV/AIDS. The major programmatic efforts addressed only the greatest number of AIDS cases, which were among gay men. Programs for women did not exist or were fragmented and oftentimes inaccessible or insensitive to women. Research studies recruited predominantly, and often times exclusively, male participants. Women's health needs and medical conditions were not carefully identified, described, or treated. This shortage of services and lack of knowledge combined with the stigma of AIDS made it very difficult for women with HIV to care for their children, some of whom were also HIV-infected. Only in recent years have women's issues and experiences begun to receive the attention and service delivery required. Unfortunately this belated response is attributable, at least in part, to the rising rate of women with HIV disease. The need for new guardians for children who have been orphaned by AIDS might be delayed if the quantity and quality of services for women were improved or even avoided altogether if effective prevention programs were offered.

As women with HIV become more seriously ill, they are confronted with concerns about the care of their children. This concern may be highlighted by long hospitalizations, prolonged near incapitation even if they are in their homes, and awareness that they are dying or near death. Bowlby advises that if a child cannot be raised by a loving parent, the psychologically sensible course of action is to identify a meaningful relative with whom the child shares some attachment and relationship as part of a broader family group.

Relatives commonly provide for a child when his or her parents are unable to do so. In recent years the private or informal arrangements have been formalized by many child welfare agencies in kinship foster care. Kinship foster care involves placing a child with a relative who has been identified, approved, licensed, and paid by a child welfare agency. This formalization has resulted in some financial and medical benefits for the caregiving relatives while subjecting a heretofore private family arrangement to agency regulation and scrutiny.

The reliance upon kinship foster care seems consistent with Bowlby's advice with regard to respecting attachment to a family. It is also congruent with the values and outlook of many cultural groups that have defined and experienced a family as a broad set of relationships involving many persons related to them by blood, marriage, or voluntary commitment. Kinship foster care has also raised a number of concerns. From the perspective of the family, there are concerns about a public agency's intrusiveness and authority around what are perceived to be private family decisions. And the financial support provided may be meager compared to the cost of caring for the child. Additional issues are (1) the assumption that kin are both qualified and committed to caring for a relative, (2) the assumption that kin are attached to the child, and (3) potential complications with regard to permanency planning.

There are also a number of troubling issues that may arise with regard to bereavement of the orphaned child who is in the custody of his or her relative:

1. In order to prevent a child's self-blame, fear, and confusion, "If at all possible the child should be allowed to talk directly with the dying loved one, so that they can share their feelings and say loving farewells" (Jewett 1982, 2). However, before and immediately after a death, well-intentioned adult family members may confuse or disturb a child by "protecting" him or her from a parent's death by excluding the child from participation in family rituals and grieving. These adults' sheltering behavior can be attributed to a lack of information or understanding, or their own death anxieties (Ellis 1989). Some researchers have claimed that children grieve and mourn as young as 6 months old and that by age 8 they are capable of offering realistic explanations of death (Ellis 1989). The child who is not included in funeral or memorial services for a parent may be left with unresolved feelings; such a state has been compared to the unsettled condition of the wife of a prisoner of war (Jewett 1982). This condition frightens the child and leads to the damaging belief that he or she has done something wrong.

For AIDS orphans in informal or foster kinship care this failure to involve the child with the dying parent or in grief rituals may be even more pronounced. The ill mother may have hidden her diagnosis and the seriousness of her illness from her children and extended family. Facing one's own death and the prospect of leaving one's children is frightening, and the realities can easily lead to denial and suppression. The stigma of AIDS may result in condemnation of the mother. Potential discrimination against the children may also incline a parent to keep her illness secret, and she may consequently fail to alert and communicate with children and family. The kin who provide care for the orphaned child may also be aware of this stigma and may feel a sense of shame or embarrassment within their community. They may also worry about how they and the children in their care will be treated by others. Because the shame around an AIDS death can be so powerful, family members may even choose not to have a funeral or memorial service. The secrecy and the stigma of AIDS complicate the grieving process for the entire family. The mourning process for the children may be burdened by increased suffering.

2. Young children see the death of a parent as a threat to their own well-being and existence. At this vulnerable time for children, special attention and focus are needed:

Young children require constant, consistent, accurate, truthful, loving support and attention. . . . During grief and mourning, the young child needs at least one adult available to him or her, one whom he or she knows, cares for and trusts. (Ellis 1989, 208)

This need highlights one of the strengths of kinship care. There is the increased likelihood that the child will be in the custody of a familiar relative, ideally one with whom the child has a trusting relationship. However, there are two potential complications. First, sometimes the life-style of the deceased mother may have estranged her from her family so that relatives have not been a positive or frequent part of the young child's life. Second, the child has lost a parent, but he or she is not the sole griever. The child's grandparent has lost a daughter, and the aunt has lost a sister. So the potentially known and trusted family members may themselves be depressed, angry, guilty, and heartbroken. There may not be a psychologically available relative able to respond supportively and attentively to the child.

3. When a child is placed with a relative there may be an assumption that the kinship relationship ensures a smooth transition. This minimizes the child's suffering associated with the death of and the separation from the parent. The child's ability to cry and feel deeply troubled at one moment and to play happily the next may confuse a caregiver. Such behavior may also support a premature assessment that the child has recovered from a parent's death. The child may have experienced some role reversal with an ill or dying parent that may have fostered a high degree of responsibility for his or her own care or considerable independence in decision making; these traits may be challenged in a new setting. A relative expecting a grateful, agreeable, respectful, and well-behaved young family member may be rudely confronted by a grieving, acting-out child:

Adults are often reluctant to respond to children in mourning—or they simply do not realize that the difficult behavior they encounter can be directly attributed to grief, and that it needs their understanding, support and attention. (Jewett 1982, vi)

The caregiver's response to the child may be further affected by the previous relationship with and judgment of the deceased parent. There may be a fear of contagion. A quiet or compliant child may not necessarily be one who has adequately mourned or even one who has begun to adjust to a new life with new relatives. Complacency may mask depression, anger, and fear as the child has not been enabled, encouraged, or allowed to grieve.

Such assumptions of comfort and adjustment may also fail to consider the multiple losses that accompany the loss of a parent and the relocation to a relative's home. Although a child may know the relative, he or she may be facing the loss of friendships and the security of the familiar. The child must overcome the insecurities associated with a new school, a new neighborhood, and new patterns and routines. These losses and disruptions may seriously affect an older child's grief process. For an adolescent, grieving may be complicated by resistance to communicating with an adult, even a family member (Rando 1984). Adolescents' ability to rely on peers and friends, rather than adults, for support and information may be compromised by their relocation and isolation from old friends. Communication with peers may also be compromised by the stigma of AIDS, which leads to an unwillingness to disclose or fully identify the stresses and losses experienced when a parent dies of AIDS. So the loss of a parent is compounded by the loss of familiar relationships and surroundings and the adolescent's potential alienation from adults (LaGrand 1989).

It is often in the best interests of an orphan that he or she be raised by a relative, assuming that a competent and committed relative is available and willing to take on this responsibility. This is the preferred placement because it preserves a family unit and places the child with someone whom he or she already knows, trusts, and loves. However, there are challenges for the grieving child, including the minimization of the child's grief or exclusion from grieving rituals, the relative's own complicated grief process that lessens the ability to tune in accurately to the child's needs, and the failure to understand the magnified loss of death, separation, and potentially troubled responses by the mourning child.

FOSTER FAMILIES

When a child whose parent has died of AIDS is placed with a nonrelated foster family, a number of outcomes may result. These outcomes are directly related to the lack of a relative who is willing and able to care for the child. Some parents with HIV who are involved in drug use, and consequently neglect their children, may be reported to child protective services. Their children will be placed in a foster home by court order. Some parents with HIV abandon their infants in the hospital, and the children are placed in foster care. Other parents become too ill to care for their children, and since no relatives can be located, the children are placed in a family foster care home. In some cases, mothers who are ill with HIV/AIDS purposely identify or work together with a child welfare agency to select and build a relationship with foster parents who will provide respite care, in some circumstances, or placement in the case of the mother's incapacity or death.

If children are identified as HIV-infected or as having AIDS, the foster home selected for placement may be a specialized foster care program that is prepared for children with HIV. These programs are located in a number of cities across the United States and have a number of features in common:

- Foster parents are recruited specifically for this program. The motivation and ability of the parents are carefully examined during an initial exploration process. In addition to parenting issues, the potential foster parents' knowledge about and comfort in caring for a child with HIV/AIDS and their ability to provide medically sensitive supervision are assessed. One specialized program found that a number of its foster parents had medical backgrounds. Almost all had some experience in caring for a close relative with a serious and terminal illness (Gurdin and Anderson 1987).

- Foster parents are specially trained at the time of initial licensing and on an ongoing basis so that they remain well informed about the medical, psychological, social, and legal information about HIV/AIDS. This training oftentimes includes grief education (Doka 1990).

- Foster parents and the children in their care are assisted by a specially trained social worker who often has a reduced caseload and works as a member of a team that may include nurses or other health workers. One program includes on its staff a chaplain who specifically assists foster parents, staff members, children, and family members with issues of grief, mourning, and spiritual concerns.

- Foster parents and the children in their care have access to a range of special services. There may be support groups for the foster parents, the children, or both, in which bereavement is an acceptable and expected topic of group discussion. Additional services may include respite care, recreation, and camp programs.

The child who has been identified as having HIV/AIDS prior to placement may have access to a specialized foster care program, in which case foster parents and highly sensitive staff members are available. This level of targeted and careful foster parent recruitment, training, and service milieu would be ideal for all children entering foster care. If an HIV-negative child is placed in a nonrelated family foster home, there is considerably less likelihood that the foster parents will be prepared for the child's AIDS-related concerns and grief.

A number of aspects of entering and continuing in foster care are not in the grieving child's best interests and in fact may be harmful. Sometimes the rapid manner in which children come into foster care, the variety of people who may have contact with them, and the assumption that children either cannot understand or do not need to know certain information result in a failure to provide even a brief orientation for already bewildered and grieving children, as in the following case.

Although foster care for the children had not been discussed with the worker or children previously, the mother told her worker that she was feeling overwhelmed and unable to care for her kids physically or emotionally at the time. She asked whether they could be placed in a foster home immediately. The worker acknowledged her desperation and attempted to locate a relative who might assist. The mother said there were no family members nearby or capable of such care. A foster home was located and the four children were transported to the home. Upon their entering the foster home, the foster mother greeted the children. Dropping to one knee she approached the youngest child, a four-year-old girl, and with the other children listening she asked the young girl whether she knew what a "foster parent" was. The girl replied she did not know. The foster mother said, " 'Foster' means friend, so I will be a friendly mother for you for a while." She then asked, "Do you know why you were brought to a foster home?" The child replied, "Yes, we need to have a place to live until our mommie gets her head together." The foster mother and worker said that was correct and began to give the children a tour of the house.

The foster parent who has the sensitivity and the knowledge to tune into the child's grief and loss can provide sensitive support by listening, asking gentle questions, encouraging the expression of feelings, accepting anger or confusion, and reframing adjustment reactions. This nurturance must take place while respecting the child's love for the parent.

There are a number of obstacles to providing sensitive care for an orphaned child. This therapeutic role of the foster parent may be limited by a scant knowledge of child development and the grief process for children. Even when the foster parent has this knowledge, it may be difficult to demonstrate sensitivity to the child's grief when he or she must respond to the needs of several children simultaneously. The grieving child's reactions to the parent's death, the separation, and the new foster home may require considerable patience, discipline, and understanding of the foster parent. There is also a need to individualize children—all kids do not have the same reaction, exhibit the same grief patterns, or respond to the same approach. Further challenging this adjustment process, the parent and children may not share a common culture and will be strangers to each other. The foster parent may also be coping with his or her own anticipatory grief if the foster child is ill (Anderson et al. 1989).

When a child is placed in a foster home, whether that home is with a relative or not, the agency's actions and decisions should be informed by a commitment to permanency planning. This planning refers to a number of guiding principles for decision making; the central one is that children need a permanent, stable home and family. This commitment became particularly crystallized in the late 1970s after studies documented the drift of children in foster care, often without the benefit of psychologically committed and legally mandated caregivers.

At the present time a number of alternatives or goals face AIDS orphans who are in the domain of child welfare: (1) return to a parent, (2) legal adoption, or, in the case of older children, (3) independent living.

Return to a Parent

Returning the child to a parent is a common discharge objective that meets the requirements for permanency planning and is congruent with the value of having children raised within their own families. For children who are orphaned by AIDS this option no longer exists. There may be an attempt to return the child to a relative who either is identified by the child or caseworker or initiates a request for guardianship of the child. For many who have not been literally orphaned there is a "functional" orphaning—a parent may be alive but completely unable to provide care for the child. This functional orphaning results from the parent's severe illness and desire to remain separate from the child because of her debilitated condition, shame about having AIDS, or belief that this is best for the child. The parent's location may be unknown and diligent search efforts by caseworkers may fail to uncover the parent's location. The parent may be in prison. The biological parent may be divorced, separated from the partner, or in a new relationship and not desiring any relationship with the child. The orphan must look to a new person to provide care.

Adoption

Particularly for younger children, but for children at all ages, adoption is consistent with permanency planning goals and provides a caregiver with appropriate legal status to care for the child. The option of adoption may be more difficult to implement for older children. Younger children may be freed for adoption, but this process often requires several years of work. In kinship care this arrangement may be particularly objectionable as grandparents or other relatives may contemplate becoming legal parents for related children by terminating the parental rights of their children, nieces, and nephews. Even when a parent has died, the option of adoption may feel inappropriate to some relatives. It may also be troubling to some children. When children are unable to mourn the death of their parents, they may find themselves unprepared to accept new parents.

Independent Living

Some children live on their own at a young age, even assuming care of younger siblings; others remain in a foster home for an extended period with the goal of independence. Not expected to be adopted and unable to return to a parent, many adolescents who go into foster care are enrolled in independent living programs. These programs are designed to assist the adolescent to prepare for life after foster care. Curriculum treats issues of daily living, shopping, check writing and financial management, employment issues, and so on. This preparation for the future is age-appropriate and parallels the tasks for all adolescents. But it may have a particular urgency for the adolescent in foster care who may not have an extended family or family to return to or look to for ongoing support during young adulthood. The programs might focus on practical necessities rather than the psychological adjustment and social reactions of teens. Adolescents in foster care who are grieving the AIDS-related loss of a parent, younger sibling, or other family member may be preoccupied with concerns about their own health and well-being. They may not share these troubles with adults or relatively unknown peers. An adolescent may need a support network but be unable to identify anyone who has gone through similar experiences of losing parents to AIDS and living in foster care. The goals of an independent living program may be too ambitious; the adolescent may be unprepared to enagage in such preparation because he or she may doubt the existence or merit of any future.

If a loss, such as the death of a parent, is expected and planned for, it may be easier for children and caregivers to respond to the challenges facing each person. For many parents dying from AIDS, however, planning for death and its aftermath may be more than they can manage. Nonetheless, some actions may be possible, including (1) planning one's funeral or memorial service and including one's children in this process, (2) identifying a person or family to care for one's children after the parent is either too ill or dead, and (3) introducing one's children to this designated family so that the children can begin to build a supportive relationship with this family. This identified family may be an unrelated foster family. One innovative program places the parent and the children with a nurturing foster parent who will become the children's caregiver upon the parent's death (Anderson 1990).

"Tell Mama I love her" was the message from the terminally ill mother in the intensive care unit to the nurse on the telephone with the foster mother of the dying woman's daughter. Mrs. B., the foster parent, had originally been assigned as a parent aide to the mother when Tina was born HIV-positive. As the relationship between the two women grew, the mother asked Mrs. B. to be Tina's godmother. And as the mother's health deteriorated, Mrs. B. became Tina's foster mother. In time, Mrs. B. became the foster parent to the mother and Tina. Now, after the mother's death, Mrs. B. is in the process of adopting Tina.

One of the most pressing questions raised in support groups for mothers with HIV is "What will happen to my children after I die? Who will care for them?" A planned process with supportive guidance and legal assistance can provide an answer to these questions and facilitate the grief process for the parent and child alike.

These arrangements that address the family's needs and concerns may be complicated by legal issues. Surrendering guardianship or voluntarily terminating one's parental rights may be unacceptable to the parent or future caregiver. Such a status may also deprive the parent of needed financial support or benefits. However, waiting until after the parent's death to settle custody may not ensure that the parent's wishes are in fact respected. An appropriate legal status to facilitate this transition that provides legal protection for the children within acceptable boundaries for concerned parties is yet to be fully defined and enacted.

To create a more flexible option, New York State enacted in June 1992 a Standby Guardian Law to allow terminally ill parents to name a proposed guardian of their children effective upon a triggering event: their physical or mental incapacity or their death. Parents who choose to appoint a standby guardian retain their parental rights, and after their death, their children avoid the waiting period and approval process that are necessary to confirm a guardian who is designated only in a will. Standby guardian designations may be accomplished through a hearing before the family or surrogate court or by a written statement, which must be filed with the court by the proposed guardian after the triggering event. Because judges have such broad discretion, however, family law attorneys suggest that written designations, which only delay the court hearing, may not assure the judge's approval of the proposed guardian (Herb 1993; Pinott 1993).

RECOMMENDATIONS

There are a number of actions that could address and perhaps lessen the trauma, if not the grief, experienced by children and families affected profoundly by AIDS. First, there should be a range of available supportive services that can sustain and bolster a parent's ability to care for her children as long as possible. In the past, there appeared to be more support services for foster families than for biological families. Foster familes need support, but biological parents also need resources to prevent or postpone the need for new guardians for their children. These services need to be culturally sensitive, accessible, comprehensive, and knowledgeable about women's health issues. Resources need to be available to extended family members as well.

Legal assistance should be available to parents with HIV. States should craft a legal status that respects ill parents' attachments to their children but grants parent-identified alternate caregivers some legal status and security.

This guardianship status might serve as an alternative to terminating parental rights.

When a parent's ability to care for a child is seriously compromised and a foster care placement is necessary, an "open" relationship or partnership with the parents has merit. A foster family can serve as a respite caregiver for a family. In this case, as a parent and a foster parent develop a relationship, the foster parent is able to care for the children, while supporting and communicating with the ill parent. The foster family is prepared eventually to adopt the child with the parent's knowledge and approval.

Finally, helping people need to be educated and supported with regard to the grieving process. Grief education for new guardians and family members does not eliminate grieving but may provide some cognitive grasp on grief that would help in the process of coping with loss and helping a child in mourning. Bereavement support groups for each family member, and all ages, may be particularly helpful for school-aged children and adolescents, in addition to adults. Guardians and professionals need to be especially attentive to the responses and fears of children.

CONCLUSION

Children whose parents have died of AIDS face a complicated grieving process. When a parent dies, children need to be reassured "that they will continue to be loved, cared for, and safe, and will remain members of the family, enjoying its protection" (Ellis 1989). This reassurance is very difficult for children orphaned by AIDS to obtain. They have little protection and considerable vulnerability. The cohesiveness of one's family, although subjected to stress prior to the parent's death, is shattered as children learn to live with new guardians. Some of these guardians may be familiar and part of one's family; others are strangers and unknown. These new families provide some opportunities for help and healing as a child grieves with a trusted relative or is supported by an attentive, well-trained foster parent.

There are also multiple risks for an ill-processed mourning response that may even threaten the stability of these new living arrangements. The new guardians of orphaned children must understand and address the child's grief and separation from a familiar home and caregiver, all within the troubling context of a stigmatized illness. Assuring children that they are not alone and helping them to cope with multiple losses will challenge the love and commitment of these new guardians.

REFERENCES

Anderson, Gary R. 1990. *Courage to Care: Responding to the Crisis of Children with AIDS*. Washington DC: Child Welfare League of America.

_____. 1990. "Creating Programs to Care for Children with HIV/AIDS." In *Courage to Care*, ed. G. R. Anderson. Washington DC: Child Welfare League of America.

Anderson, Gary R., and Phyllis Gurdin. "Children with AIDS: Permanency Planning Issues." Unpublished.

Anderson, Gary R., Phyllis Gurdin, and Ann Thomas. 1989. "Dual Disenfranchisement: Foster Parenting Children with AIDS." In *Disenfranchised Grief*, ed. K. J. Doka. Lexington, MA: Lexington Books.

Bowlby, John. 1967. *Maternal Care and Mental Health*. New York: Schocken Books.

Doka, Kenneth J. 1990. "Grief Education: Educating About Death for Life." In *Courage to Care*, ed. G. R. Anderson. Washington DC: Child Welfare League of America.

Ellis, Richard R. 1989. "Young Children: Disenfranchised Grievers." In *Disenfranchised Grief*, ed. K. J. Doka. Lexington, MA: Lexington Books.

Gurdin, Phyllis, and Gary R. Anderson. 1987. "Quality Care for Ill Children: AIDS Specialized Foster Family Homes." *Child Welfare* 66:291–302.

Herb, Alice. 1993. "The New York State Standby Guardianship Law: A New Option for Terminally Ill Parents." In *A Death in the Family: Orphans of the HIV Epidemic*, ed. Carol Levine, 87–93. New York: United Hospital Fund.

Jewett, Claudia. 1982. *Helping Children Cope with Separation and Loss*. Boston: The Harvard Common Press.

LaGrand, Louis. 1989. "Youth and the Disenfranchised Breakup." In *Disenfranchised Grief*, ed. K. J. Doka. Lexington, MA: Lexington Books.

Pinott, Mildred. 1993. "Custody and Placement: The Legal Issues." In *A Death in the Family: Orphans of the HIV Epidemic*, ed. Carol Levine, 75–84. New York: United Hospital Fund.

Rando, Therese. 1984. *Grief, Dying, and Death*. Champaign, IL: Research Press.

9

Programs for Children
and Adolescents

Diane Grodney

INTRODUCTION

The needs of healthy children and adolescents who are surviving parental death from AIDS have not received sufficient programmatic attention.[1] These young orphans have usually grown up in communities blighted by drug use, violence, poverty, and racism. One study (Draimin et al. 1992) found that these adolescents had experienced an average of four major losses in the two years prior to the parent's death from AIDS. Over 80 percent had experienced at least one loss. Thus, although these children may seem invisible, the multiple traumas they have faced and their vulnerability make it imperative that we develop programs that attend to their needs.

Originally, the plan for this chapter was to describe bereavement programs around the country which serve children and adolescents who have lost significant others to AIDS. However, as such programs are limited, scattered, and in the earliest stages of development, attention was turned to services within the New York–New Jersey metropolitan area. This region has the largest number of HIV-infected women and children and surviving minors in the United States. The programs discussed here were selected because their planners have been particularly creative in reducing barriers to service and promoting a flexible approach to service delivery that recognizes, supports, and honors clients' values, beliefs, and life-styles.

Although three of the four programs are affiliated with medical centers, the responsibility for providing services to these children and adolescents cannot, and should not, remain primarily within hospital settings. These children and their newly reconstituted families need services located in their own communities and linked to their natural support systems (e.g., schools, religious organizations, and community centers).

The main objectives of this chapter are to provide an in-depth review of four programs and to offer guidance to professionals who are considering developing such programs within their own organizations. The chapter is divided into brief program descriptions and clinical issues, including illustrative vignettes; treatment approaches, including group therapy, family therapy, and community interventions; and recommendations.

BRIEF PROGRAM DESCRIPTIONS

Well Children in AIDS Families Project, Beth Israel Medical Center, New York City

The Well Children in AIDS Families Project was developed by Beth Israel Medical Center (BIMC) in 1987. BIMC has approximately 1,900 adult patients registered in the Infectious Disease Clinic and at least 90 children in the Pediatric Infectious Disease Clinic. The Well Children in AIDS Families Project was designed to address the needs of children who are HIV-negative themselves but are living in families where a parent or sibling either is HIV-infected, has AIDS, or has died of AIDS. For the most part, the children who have come to the program have had a parent who is ill or who has died from AIDS. Approximately 40 percent of the work is around the children's bereavement needs.

Originally, the project existed under the auspices of the Department of Psychiatry. Referrals were sparse when it was housed in this location. Several changes enhanced the program's visibility and accessibility. First, the program was relocated to the Pediatric Outpatient Clinic, where the social worker became a familiar figure to the healthy children who attended the clinic with their ill siblings. The child was also able to interact with the HIV social workers on a more informal basis. Subsequently, the HIV social workers referred adult patients to him for consultation concerning their healthy children. He was able to destigmatize the service to the parents by explaining that many normal children exhibit behavioral changes when experiencing family crises. The medical center also began to publicize the program widely. As a result of these changes, the program became quite popular.

Beth Israel has also begun to form partnerships with service providers in the community, such as the Jewish Board of Family & Children's Services (JBFCS), which has a long history of providing community-based services to families and children. JBFCS clinicians are invited to the hospital to see prospective clients prior to discharge. It is hoped that the pretherapy connection will facilitate successful referrals.

The Family Place, Children's Hospital, Newark, New Jersey

The Family Place is a multifaceted, community-based social service program. It offers intensive case management; respite care; individual, family, and group counseling; bereavement counseling; substance abuse assessment, intervention, and referral services; support groups for healthy siblings; social/recreational activities; and foster parent training. Any member of a family that is impacted by HIV/AIDS is eligible for service. "Family" is broadly defined to include biological, extended, foster, and adoptive families. The Family Place responds to the needs of the family as defined by the family and provides linkages with appropriate resources.

Although the Family Place is the community outreach component of the New Jersey Children's Hospital AIDS Program (CHAP), the two programs share only a small number of cases. The Family Place provides case management services to 115 families under a grant from the State's Division of Youth & Family Services. It also provides mental health services to another 186 individuals. The Family Place has earned significant credibility within the Newark community and reports no difficulty obtaining referrals. The most frequently encountered obstacle has been securing reliable transportation for the children.

AIDS Programming, Bronx Lebanon Hospital, New York City

The South Bronx is an epicenter of the AIDS epidemic. Bronx Lebanon Hospital currently has 2,300 patients enrolled in the Infectious Disease Clinic. As the Social Work Department began working with adults with HIV/AIDS the question arose, What is going to happen to the children in these families? The Family Outreach Program was created in response to this concern. The only eligibility criterion is that there be an HIV-infected adult in the family. The Family Outreach Program is available to both inpatients and outpatients.

The Family Outreach Program has two components—a program that provides case management for children of HIV-infected parents and a program for new guardians. The case management program serves children and their infected parents by focusing on concrete needs, disclosure and custody determination. The new guardians program targets reconstructed families after the death of the infected individual. The programs are based upon a model of continuum of care in which patients are eligible for services from the moment of diagnosis onward. Social workers treat the primary patients until their death and see the newly reconstructed families as long as there is a defined need.

Social workers at Bronx Lebanon Hospital have been more successful in engaging patients during hospitalization than after discharge. Although parents with AIDS have been responsive to the Family Outreach Program, newly reconstituted families have not returned for services after the parents died. Treatment drop-out may occur because the family moves away or because relatives do not wish to rekindle the sad memories associated with the hospital. To reach a greater number of families in need of assistance, recruitment for the new guardians program will target families throughout the borough.

Community Consultation Center, Henry Street Settlement, New York City

Located on the Lower East Side of Manhattan, Henry Street Settlement serves a community that has one of the highest rates of AIDS in the United States. Henry Street's mental health component is the Community Consultation Center (CCC). CCC first became involved in AIDS in 1979, when a staff member died of what was originally thought to be tuberculosis but was later understood to have been AIDS. By 1982, CCC discovered that several clients were symptomatic with HIV and others had family members who were ill or dying.

In 1982, Henry Street was designated by the New York City Department of Mental Health as the service provider for people with AIDS and their families in the Lower East Side. Despite extensive outreach efforts, few clients initially came for help. Several plausible explanations for the lack of successful referrals were considered. First, it was recognized that families who had experienced a death from AIDS shielded themselves with "a blanket of silence." Secrecy arose out of a profound need to preserve dignity and self-respect and to defend against social ostracization, stigmatization, and discrimination. However, the silence also negatively impacted the families' and community's ability to cope with the epidemic. A second reason for the lack of successful referrals was related to the way in which referrals were made. The health care professionals referring families to CCC had not helped patients redefine their needs within a mental health framework. Thus, clients did not understand the rationale for the referral and continued to see their needs solely within a medical, rather than a psychosocial context.

In 1988, a local guidance counselor sought help from Henry Street for several children who had experienced recent familial deaths and were misbehaving in school. Because of the secrecy surrounding these families, it was hypothesized that the deaths may have been from AIDS. The school asked CCC to develop bereavement services in the school, and despite a lack of funding, three groups were started. By utilizing a natural helping system in the community (i.e., schools), CCC was able to reach out to the children in a nonstigmatizing way. Parents readily gave consent for their children to attend the groups. Subsequently, CCC staff was able to reach out to the families successfully and engage them in intergenerational reparation work. Henry Street now provides a combination of individual, group and family therapy for families and children affected by AIDS.

CLINICAL ISSUES: EMOTIONAL REACTIONS

The following section focuses on the range of emotional reactions experienced by children and adolescents orphaned as a result of AIDS, issues specific to adolescent survivors, and custody planning and termination.

Healthy children and adolescents who have survived losses to AIDS are at great emotional, developmental, and behavioral risk. Childrens' reactions are just what one might expect—fear of death, anger, feelings of loss and abandonment, and suicidal ideation and gestures. This section will consider children's and adolescents' reactions by offering illustrative case vignettes. Clinical issues related to saying good-bye and disclosing the secret of AIDS will also be addressed.

Fear of Death

A child and her mother were seen for bereavement work after the death of the father. The mother and child were HIV-negative.

During one session, the mother reported that the child was having trouble sleeping. I thought she might be afraid she was going to die. When this was suggested, and the child acknowledged the fear, the youngster and mother were reassured that many children have a similar reaction to the death of a parent. (McKelvy 1992)

Anger

Children who are old enough to understand the ways in which HIV is transmitted may be extraordinarily disappointed in and angry at the parent for engaging in the behavior. "My mother was sexually active? What was she thinking about?"

Guilt

Many children are guilt-ridden and feel they have caused their mother to get sick.

"I was a bad boy; I didn't listen to her." Children may believe they are responsible. Adolescents may admit, "You know, I gave her a really hard time, I was always hanging out, I wouldn't come home." It's very easy to get kids to accept the guilt. Mothers may say to children, "You're killing me; you're making me sick." Unfortunately, even though the parents don't really mean it, the children do not forget it. (Pincus-Strom 1992)

Loss and Abandonment

Understandably, children experience a great deal of anxiety about who will care for them if their mother dies. Often, this is not the first loss or death the child has experienced. The family may have been evicted any number of times. The mother may have had a drug habit. The children may have been placed in foster care for a period of time. The death of the mother tends to reevoke all the prior losses and creates a deep sense of abandonment in children.

Suicidal Ideation and Gestures

Children have also been known to have suicidal ideation after the death of the parent. Sometimes the ideation is clearly an identification with the parent who has died from AIDS.

A teenage girl was admitted to the Hospital with pelvic inflammatory disease. Basically, she said to me: "My mother died, my father died, my brother died, I want to be with them and I'm going to go get it too." Unfortunately, I could never get her into treatment. (McKelvy 1992)

Suicidal gestures may take other forms:

I see a 14–year-old Puerto Rican boy whose parents died of AIDS. He was abused by them during his childhood. He rides between the subway cars barely holding onto the sides, and once he jumped out of a second story window. Suicidal ideation and gestures walk hand-in-hand in his daily life. He is a very tough kid who is difficult to engage. He comes in for sessions, but he still acts on his impulses. He is full of rage. He'll say, "I hate Blacks and I hate Jews. And you're white and you don't know shit." In his mind, he's annihilated just about everybody. We've gotten through some of the negative reactions to me because he's been able to verbalize them. (McKelvy 1992)

Sometimes, suicidal ideation is a way of expressing a wish for reunion with the parent.

One of the most difficult interviews I ever participated in was with a woman who had just given us permission to tell her children she had AIDS. We knew she had little time left. Her children were in different foster homes. She wanted to see them each before she died. When the 10–year-old came in with his social worker, we sat in my office and I prepared him for what he would see. When we went up to the room he asked his mother, "Mommy, are you going to die?" His mother could hardly speak, she was so sick. And he said, "Mommy, if you die I'm going to go and kill myself because I don't want to live without you and I want to be with you in heaven." We came back to my office and talked about life without Mommy and how it can still be worth living. His social worker was in tears, and this poor little boy sat on her lap sobbing. It's not unusual for children to believe in a reunion in heaven, but this belief can result in repeating the high-risk behavior. (Pincus-Strom 1992)

Saying Good-Bye

"Social agencies need to come to terms with their own irrational fears about AIDS to help children have positive contact with dying parents and help them to ask needed questions" (Demb 1989, 243). The practitioners interviewed agreed that it is important for a child to have a final visit with his or her mother. Of course, these clinicians would only take a child to the parent's bedside if it were the child's wish and if a visit were in the best interest of the child. An assessment would have to be based on the child's age and emotional state and the parent's emotional and physical condition.

Disclosing the Secret of AIDS

Stigma, based on ignorance and fear, continues to affect families with HIV infection and AIDS. Parents may hide their HIV status from children to preserve the dignity and self-respect of the family, protect the child from social ostracization, and/or prevent discrimination in housing, employment, and medical care. Parents may also refuse to tell children of their HIV status out of shame, self-hatred, fear of rejection, or concern that the child will insist on giving up his or her own life to take care of the parent. In treating these families, it is imperative to know whether or not the children are aware of the parent's diagnosis.

One of the most difficult tasks a mother can face is telling her child she has AIDS and may die. It is advisable for her to wait to disclose that information until she has begun to manage her own feelings. Often, the child already knows the truth but feels unable to speak about it without the parent's permission. If there has been no discussion of the parent's illness, the child cannot begin anticipatory grief work. If the parent decides that the children should know, program clinicians can help the family through the process of disclosure and anticipatory mourning:

It's very hard to work with a child who does not know the parent's diagnosis and many parents are reluctant to tell. In such cases, the work with the parent can focus on disclosure, and the work with the child can be around having an ill parent. In most but not all cases, disclosure ultimately takes place. We leave it to the parent to give consent for us to assist with disclosure. Many of the parents just can't do it; it's too painful. And they'll ask, "Will you do it? Will you tell my child?" And we'll say, "OK, we'll have a family meeting, and if you can't do it, I'll do it for you. And then we can deal with it together." (Pincus-Strom 1992)

CLINICAL ISSUES: ADOLESCENT SURVIVORS

The turmoil, regressive pulls, reckless behavior, and depression charac-teristic of the adolescence phase are further complicated by the actual loss of a parent (Demb 1989). Adolescent survivors are at great risk for engaging in acting-out behaviors such as unsafe sex, dropping out of school, violence, drugs, and other criminal activity. The risks for adolescents who have parents with HIV/AIDS are compounded when they also have younger siblings who are infected or who have died.

In one of our families the mother and three of four siblings are infected. Our biggest concern is over what will happen to the healthy child when everyone else dies. It's a tremendous burden. We know we may not see the impact of such extensive loss until three, four, or five years down the line. That's why we need to advise the parental surrogates that there could be serious repercussions for the child in the years to come. (Pincus-Strom 1992)

Often an adolescent will become the parentified child and assume re-sponsibility for the ill parent and healthy or sick siblings.

We've seen many children drop out of school to take care of their parents and siblings. In one case, the parent was heterosexually infected, and did not find out her HIV status until she gave birth to a sick child. The child not only had HIV, but also had cerebral palsy and a number of other conditions. He was not expected to live very long. There were two older daughters from a previous relationship. The older daughter got married and moved to Pennsylvania. The second daughter had just started college. She dropped out and stayed home to take care of her infected mother and very sick brother. The brother lived for three years. This never would have happened if it were not for the care his sister gave him. When the boy died, the mother went into a deep depression and died shortly thereafter. This young woman was our biggest concern because in addition to the deaths of her mother and brother, she stood to lose her housing, she had no job, she had given up school, and she had nothing. Her entire life had been devoted to caring for her mother and brother. (Pincus-Strom 1992)

CLINICAL ISSUES: CUSTODY

Fortunately, the children in these programs have usually had an imme-diate or extended family member who was willing and able to care for them after their mothers died. Few children had to be referred to the foster care system. There is grave concern for siblings who have to be separated after the death of their mother.

One of our "successful" cases was a mother of two children, ages 13 and 3. We had been working with her for quite a while on custody determination. She was very sick. She had one sister who was an HIV-infected drug user and another sister who was healthy. The healthy sister was willing to take the children but suddenly had to move to Texas because of her husband's job.

After working with the mother for a while, we learned that the 3 year-old was not her biological child. She had taken him in as a foster child when he was 4 days old. It was agreed that she would adopt him. However, the mother became too ill to continue the adoption process. We couldn't get this boy to Texas to see whether or not his aunt would even be interested in adopting him because a foster child is not allowed to leave the state. We could get the girl there, but we knew that if she lost her brother, on top of losing her mother, she would be completely torn up by it. The daughter had essentially raised this child by herself because her mother was so ill. The two children were very close.

We worked hard to prevent this little boy from having to be placed in foster care. We were able to get the aunt to visit from Texas and she decided to adopt the boy. The children moved to Texas together. This was the best possible outcome for them. (Pincus-Strom 1992)

CLINICAL ISSUES: TERMINATION OF TREATMENT

Surviving children frequently suffer many losses including parent(s), sibling(s), school, home, neighborhood, friends, and social supports. Considering the prevalence of loss and abandonment in these children's lives, termination of treatment needs to be carefully addressed. Several clinicians have found that children and their families will not initiate ending on their own. However, the clinician may begin the termination process when there are a remission in symptoms, stabilization in family structure, and lack of emotional upheaval. Although the case may be closed administratively, the door usually remains open.

TREATMENT APPROACHES

The clinicians in these programs use creative, culturally sensitive, and flexible approaches in their work. Such sensitivity is of paramount importance because poor families, families of color, and families affected by AIDS frequently feel alienated from mental health providers. Clinicians have pointed to the stabilization of families with AIDS as one of their most important goals.

Although family and group interventions are particularly valuable for people whose lives are touched by AIDS, clients may not wish to participate in these modalities. Some children may need the special attention provided by individual therapy. Group treatment may be inappropriate for adolescents who relate poorly to peers or who find verbal exploration of feelings too threatening. In these situations, it may be valuable to begin the child or adolescent in individual therapy and move toward group intervention later.

Further, it may not be logistically, structurally, or emotionally feasible to bring family members together for therapy (McKelvy 1992).

This section focuses on the use of family, group, and community interventions. Innovative approaches such as art, audio/videotaping, and sports will also be discussed since verbal expression of anticipatory grief and mourning may be too overwhelming, too painful, or beyond the developmental capabilities of the child.

Group Therapy

Group therapy is widely recognized as an effective method of intervention for grieving adults (Vinogradov and Yalom 1989; Yalom and Vinogradov 1988). Bereavement support groups are also known to help children through the processes of identification, universalization, and normalization (Zambelli and DeRosa 1992). Because of the stigma and social isolation associated with AIDS, groups are especially important to people grieving losses from the disease. Each of the programs described in this chapter is using groups extensively or planning for them. For example, Bronx Lebanon is planning a group for new guardians, a group for children, and a group for adolescents. This section focuses on implementing and leading groups for children and adolescents.

In 1992, the Family Place conducted three groups for siblings who were not HIV-infected themselves but had dying family members.

There was a time when it seemed that nearly all the members of one of the siblings' groups had someone in the family who was near end stage. The children made "get well" cards in the group. The next week, when a group member's sibling died, the children in the group went to the family's home with our social worker. This family had very little social contact. It was wonderful for them to know that there was a group of children who were thinking of them and caring about them. The children who visited the family experienced an important breakthrough in denial. (Kreibick 1992)

Some children find it too painful to talk after the death has occurred, and artwork is used at the Family Place to facilitate self-expression in the groups. Physical exercise is used to help hyperactive or acting-out children express their feelings. The siblings groups also offer substance abuse prevention. As these children grow up in families and communities marked by extensive substance abuse, they are at very high risk for becoming involved in drugs. The substance abuse prevention approach used in the groups is not necessarily to talk about drugs per se, but to discuss alternatives, develop decision-making skills, and enhance self-esteem.

In 1988, at the request of a local school, Henry Street Settlement implemented several school-based bereavement groups for children who were experiencing difficulty after the death of a parent. Clinicians at CCC hypothesized that the deaths may have resulted from AIDS, drug abuse, or violence. Although they could not be certain of the cause of parental death, each of the children had been traumatized, and the clinicians believed that the common experience of loss would bond group members. Many of the children's parents had, in fact, died of AIDS. Since group leaders did not know whether the children were aware of their parents' cause of death, AIDS could not necessarily be discussed directly.

Each year, group composition is determined by the children's needs. At first, groups were created according to natural constellations of children. For example, when four children from one family were referred, the siblings were kept together and joined with two siblings from another family to form a group. A second group was created for other unrelated children.

Later, age was used as a criterion for membership. There was a group for younger children (first through third grade) and a group for older children (fourth through sixth grade). It was later found that younger and older children were of valuable assistance to one another when placed in the same group.

During one year, groups were organized according to stage of grief. One group was developed for children who were experiencing anticipatory grief; a second group was designed for children who were living with a chronically or terminally ill parent; and a third group was designed for children whose parent had already died. The group leaders now feel that the overarching experience of living through a traumatic experience of loss bonds the children in a way which transcends other differences.

In addition to encouraging discussion of a wide range of feelings, group leaders also utilize a variety of nonverbal methods, such as artwork, which helps the children reveal themes of death and disruption in family life; letter writing to the deceased or dying parent; and audiotaping.

The groups have been operating for the past four years. Children may remain in a group as long as they attend the school. One sign of the groups' success is that members encourage other children who they know are grieving to join the groups.

It may be difficult to implement in-person groups in rural communities and sections of the country where people with AIDS are geographically dispersed. Telephone groups have been used extensively by Lori Wiener, Pediatric Branch, National Cancer Institute, National Institutes of Health. These highly confidential groups provide an opportunity for acceptance, support, self-disclosure and sharing of mutual fears and concerns. The people with AIDS and significant others who participate in the telephone groups would otherwise be isolated because of the stigma associated with the disease and the lack of adequate support networks in their geographic communities (Wiener et al. 1991).

Family Therapy

Most of these programs provide a predominantly family-centered approach to helping. "Family" is flexibly defined and may refer to an intact nuclear family, a lesbian couple, a single-parent family, an aunt or uncle, or any adult who is significant to the child. The Family Place and Henry Street Settlement CCC frequently conduct sessions in the clients' homes. Often, these home visits are conducted by teams of clinicians. Depending on the identified needs of a particular family, the worker may see several generations of the family at once or may meet with smaller subsets of family members. This section describes various family interventions including illustrative vignettes.

Family stabilization and empowerment are the primary goals of treatment at the Family Place:

There was one family which had seven deaths in one year. When the cat died, it was the final straw. I conducted three family therapy sessions. In the third session, the mother brought in some of her nieces and nephews whose mother had died. The session took place in the clients' living room and included sixteen adults and five young children. I went in without an agenda because I wanted them to tell me what they wanted. They gathered together the last ten years of photographs and showed me each person who had died. It was the first time they were together as a family since the deaths had occurred. They talked about the anger they felt and wept over their losses. (Kreibick 1992)

A family intervention at Bronx Lebanon Hospital may take the form of helping the parent decide whether or not to tell the child about the parent's illness or impending death. If the decision is made to tell the child, the parent is assisted in considering when and how to do so. The social worker helps clear the way for the child to see the parent and supports the child in coping with the visit. Social workers often take photographs of the parent and child together and help create scrapbooks and videotapes. These visits and memorabilia are important to the child's grief work and help the child keep the memory of the parent alive.

Once the children are involved in the Henry Street Settlement bereavement groups, clinicians begin to engage the parent with AIDS or the surrogate parent. This intergenerational reparation model was developed by Florence Samperi, Associate Director of the CCC, who strongly believes that kinship placement may collapse when past conflicts and traumas have not been adequately addressed. Although children in these families have certainly experienced significant familial conflict, the parents have also faced similar experiences within their own families of origin. The intergenerational model challenges the clinician to work simultaneously with three generations: the grandparent/surrogate parent, the parent with AIDS, and the child. The aim of reparation work is to interrupt the transmission of negative attitudes and feelings across the generations.

Two siblings, ages 8 and 11, whose mother was ill with AIDS, were angry and acting out in school and home. The children were enraged at their mother for being sick and for past neglect. In turn, the mother was hostile and ambivalent toward her own mother, who had abandoned her at a very early age. At times, she was adamant that her mother not receive custody of her children after her death. The social agencies involved misunderstood this woman's anger and sadness and proceeded to make custody arrangements that excluded the grandmother.

CCC staff intervened by first convening a meeting of all the agencies involved to clarify the mother's ambivalence and develop a consistent set of responses to this woman's erratic requests. The grandmother's involvement was positively reframed and the negative alliance with the mother against the grandmother was resolved. This meeting initiated the beginning of the three-generational reconnection process. While the two children were being helped in the group, the staff simultaneously intervened to help their mother deal with issues of abandonment by her own mother. After the mother was given the chance to express her anger and sadness, she was able to understand the situation that led to her abandonment. Similarly, she was now able to understand her children's angry feelings toward her for abandoning them through illness and death.

The staff saw the grandmother alone and also saw her jointly with her daughter. The grandmother admitted to abandoning her daughter and shared her guilt and regret. This process freed the grandmother to truly reclaim her daughter and to care for her until her death. Reconciliation between the generations settled the issue of guardianship of the children, who were able to acknowledge their wish to live with the grandmother without feeling disloyal to their mother. (Samperi 1992)

Community Interventions

Community-level intervention is critical in the AIDS crisis. The Family Place hires community residents to provide outreach to families. This approach has helped the program to engage effectively clients who might otherwise remain disaffiliated. As knowledgeable residents of the community, the outreach workers are also able to keep track of homeless families and families in crisis. The community workers have helped the program develop visibility, credibility, and respect within an impoverished and dangerous neighborhood.

Social workers at Bronx Lebanon Hospital were instrumental in organizing the Bronx Coalition for Children, which is an organization that comprises agencies serving families with AIDS. The goal of the Coalition is to influence legislation, develop programs, and educate professionals and patients. Two major conferences were sponsored by the Coalition. In April 1991, "Children of Loss" was attended by more than 300 professionals. The following April, "Power to the Parents," a conference designed for parents and professionals, featured an HIV-infected woman who described her experiences with her children. The presentation was followed by a series of workshops on topics such as disclosure and children's reactions, which were co-led by a parent and a professional. About 80 parents attended.

RECOMMENDATIONS

To enhance accessibility of services, programs should consider:

- Implementing a short, humane intake process;
- Providing continuity of care from diagnosis through stabilization of the reconstructed family;
- Utilizing a psychoeducational approach that underscores the normality of children's responses to parental death;
- Providing strong, consistent, genuine outreach efforts that may be successfully implemented by community residents;
- Locating services in the client's communities.

Individual, group, family and community interventions should be available. There should be a careful assessment of the complex psychosocial variables involved in clients' lives before selecting the modality of intervention. Clinicians can help children with anticipatory grief work by facilitating a final visit with the parent; helping the parent disclose the illness, if appropriate; and collecting memorabilia so the child can preserve the memory of the parent. While bereavement groups can provide effective supports for children, adolescents, or adults, nonverbal techniques frequently facilitate expression of painful feelings and conflicts surrounding parental death.

Family stabilization is the most important goal of treatment. The program's definition of "family" must be flexible enough to adapt to a wide variety of life-styles. Family sessions may be successfully conducted by a team of clinicians in the clients' homes. Planning for care of the child after the parent's death is of critical importance if foster care placements are to be avoided. Intergenerational family therapy can help repair relationships, interrupt the transmission of negative attitudes across generations, and prevent collapse of custodial arrangements.

Programs can raise consciousness within their communities by:

- Educating teachers, clergy, funeral directors, professionals, and so on;
- Advocating for legislation that supports children and families;
- Developing partnerships with other agencies to support and empower one another.

Workers also need support from their agencies. This can take a variety of forms, including consistent, responsive supervision and in-service training; development of strong, effective teams that are available for consultation on an informal and a formal basis; and time off to grieve. Although this work is complex, labor-intensive, and emotionally demanding, it is also profoundly rewarding.

NOTE

1. The author is deeply grateful to the following individuals, who have generously contributed their time, expertise and insight to the creation of this chapter: Renee Warshofsky, Director of Social Services, Beth Israel Medical Center, New York City; Lockhart McKelvy, Social Worker, Well Children in AIDS Families Project, Beth Israel Medical Center, New York City; Theresa Kreibick, Program Director, The Family Place, Children's Hospital, Newark, New Jersey; Diane Pincus-Strom, Associate Director, Department of Social Work, AIDS Programming, Staff Development and Education, Bronx Lebanon Hospital, New York City; and Larraine Ahto, Director and Chief Administrator for Mental Health Services, Community Consultation Center (CCC), Henry Street Settlement, Florence L. Samperi, Associate Director of CCC and Director of Training, Henry Street Settlement, and Lela Charney, Director of AIDS Services, Henry Street Settlement, New York City.

REFERENCES

Adams-Greenly, Margaret, Tania Siminiski-Maher, Noreen McGowan, and Paul Meyers. 1986. "A Group Program for Helping Siblings of Children with Cancer." *Journal of Psychosocial Oncology* 4:55–67.

Demb, J. 1989. "Clinical Vignette: Adolescent Survivors of Parents with AIDS." *Family Systems Medicine* 7:339–343.

Draimin, Barbara, Jan Hudis, and Jose Segura. 1992. "The Mental Health Needs of Well Adolescents in Families with AIDS." City of New York, Human Resources Administration, Division of AIDS Services, Planning and Community Affairs Department.

Kreibick, Theresa. 1992. Interview (28 September).

McKelvy, Lock. 1992. Interview (11 January).

Pincus-Strom, Diane. 1992. Interview (30 September).

Rounds, K. A., M. J. Galinsky, and L.S. Stevens. 1991. "Linking Persons with AIDS in Rural Communities: The Telephone Support Group." *Social Work* 31:13–18.

Samperi, Florence. 1991. "AIDS and Survivorship: A Three Generational Approach." Paper presented at the First International AIDS Conference on Biopsychosocial Aspects of HIV Infection, Amsterdam, Netherlands, September 24.

———. 1992. Interview (30 December).

Vinogradov, Sophia, and Irvin D. Yalom. 1989. *A Concise Guide to Group Psychotherapy.* Washington, DC: American Psychiatric Press.

Wiener, Lori S., Elizabeth Dupont Spencer, Robert Davidson, and Cynthia Fair. 1993. "National Telephone Support Groups: A New Avenue Toward Psychosocial Support for HIV-Infected Children and Their Families." *Social Work with Groups* 16:55–71.

Yalom, Irvin D., and Sophia Vinogradov. 1988. "Bereavement Groups: Techniques and Themes." *International Journal of Group Psychotherapy* 38:419–445.

Zambelli, Grace C., and Arnold P. DeRosa. 1992. "Bereavement Support Groups for School-Age Children: Theory, Intervention, and Case Example." *American Journal of Orthopsychiatry* 62:484–493.

Appendix: Resource Guide

There are very few resources for this specific population of children. However, the following selected list of AIDS organizations, child welfare organizations, and professional groups may be useful in obtaining information and referrals.

NATIONAL ORGANIZATIONS

Child Welfare League of America
440 1st Street, NW
Suite 310
Washington, DC 20001–2085
(202) 638–2952

National Black Child Development Institute
1023 15th Street, NW
Suite 600
Washington, DC 20005
(202) 387–1281

National Minority AIDS Council
300 I Street, NE
Suite 400
Washington, DC 20002
(202) 544–1076

National Institute of Child Health and Human Development
9000 Rockville Pike
Bethesda, MD 20892
(301) 496–5133

American Bar Association
Center on Children and the Law
1800 M Street, NW
Suite 200 South
Washington, DC 20036
(202) 331–2250

Family and Child Services
929 L Street, NW
Washington, DC 20001
(202) 289–1510

National Pediatric HIV Resource Center
15 South 9th Street
Newark, NJ 07107
(201) 268–8251

CDC National AIDS Clearinghouse
P.O. Box 6003
Rockville, MD 20849–6003
(800) 458–5231

Compassionate Friends
P.O. Box 3696
Oakbrook, IL 60522–3696
(708) 990–0010

Big Brothers/Big Sisters of America
230 North 13th Street
Philadelphia, PA 19107
(215) 567–7000

The Rainbow Connection
477 Hannah Branch Road
Burnsville, NC 28714
(704) 675–5909

The Good Grief Program
Judge Baker Children's Center
295 Longwood Avenue
Boston, MA 02115
(617) 232-8390, ext. 2111

Association for the Care of Children's Health
7910 Woodmont Avenue
Suite 300
Bethesda, MD 20814–3015
(301) 654–6549

National Association of People with AIDS
1423 K Street, NW
8th Floor
Washington, DC 20005
(202) 898–0414

National Association of Social Workers
P.O. Box 92180
Washington, DC 20090–2180
(202) 408–8600

TRAINING AND EDUCATION

Association for Death Education and Counseling
638 Prospect Avenue
Hartford, CT 06105–4298
(203) 232–4825

National Center for Death Education
Mount Ida College
777 Dedham Street
Newton Centre, MA 02159.
(617) 969–7000, ext. 249

BIBLIOGRAPHIES AND RESOURCE GUIDES

AIDS and Ethics [annotated bibliography]. (Washington, DC: National Association of Social Workers, n.d.).

"Bibliographies," in Nancy Boyd Webb's *Helping Bereaved Children: A Handbook for Practitioners* (New York: Guilford Press, 1993), p. 294.

"Bibliography," in Gary Anderson, ed., *Courage to Care: Responding to the Crisis of Children with AIDS* (Washington, DC: Child Welfare League of America, 1990), p. 369.

"Directory and Resources," in Gary Anderson, ed., *Courage to Care: Responding to the Crisis of Children with AIDS* (Washington, DC: Child Welfare League of America, 1990), p. 345.

Family AIDS Resource Guide, Revised 1992 (New York: New York City Department of Health). Available through the New York City AIDS Program Services' HIV Resource Library at (212) 788–4283 or through AIDS Media and Materials at (212) 285–4631.

HIV AIDS Resources for Adolescents (New York: AIDS and Adolescent Network of New York, 1993). Available through the Network, (212) 925–6675.

Living with AIDS: A Guide to Resources in New York City, Third Edition (New York: Gay Men's Health Crisis, 1993).

"Resource Guide," in Carol Levine, ed., *A Death in the Family: Orphans of the HIV Epidemic* (New York: The United Hospital Fund, 1993), p. 124.

"Selected Bibliography," in Carol Levine, ed., *A Death in the Family: Orphans of the HIV Epidemic* (New York: The United Hospital Fund, 1993), p. 154.

Index

About the Contributors

GARY R. ANDERSON, Ph.D, is associate professor at Hunter College School of Social Work.

ESTHER CHACHKES, M.S.W, is the director of social work at New York University Hospital.

BARBARA O. DANE, D.S.W., is associate professor at the New York University School of Social Work.

KENNETH J. DOKA, Ph.D, is professor of gerontology at the College of New Rochelle, New York.

BARBARA FREUND, Ph.D., is a lecturer at New York University and is in private practice in New York City.

DIANE GRODNEY, Ph.D., is associate director of field work at the New York University School of Social Work.

REGINA JENNINGS, M.S.W., is a psychotherapist in private practice in New York City.

PENELOPE JOHNSON-MOORE, D.S.W., is assistant director of the Onsite School Program at the Hillside Eastern Queens Mental Health Center and adjunct professor at the New York University School of Social Work.

CAROL LEVINE, M.A., is executive director of The Orphan Project and former executive director of the Citizens Commission on AIDS for New York City and Northern New Jersey.

LUCRETIA J. PHILLIPS, D.S.W., is the assistant dean of the branch campus at New York University School of Social Work.

KATHLEEN ROMANO, Ph.D., is a psychologist at the department of Family Medicine, Montefiore Medical Center/Albert Einstein College of Medicine.

KAROLYNN SIEGEL, Ph.D., is the director of social work research at Memorial Sloan Kettering Hospital.

LUIS H. ZAYAS, Ph.D., is psychosocial coordinator at the department of Family Medicine, Montefiore Medical Center/Albert Einstein College of Medicine, and is also affiliated with the Hispanic Research Center, Fordham University.

ISBN 0-86569-220-3

HARDCOVER BAR CODE